Thymus

Edited by Nima Rezaei

Published in London, United Kingdom

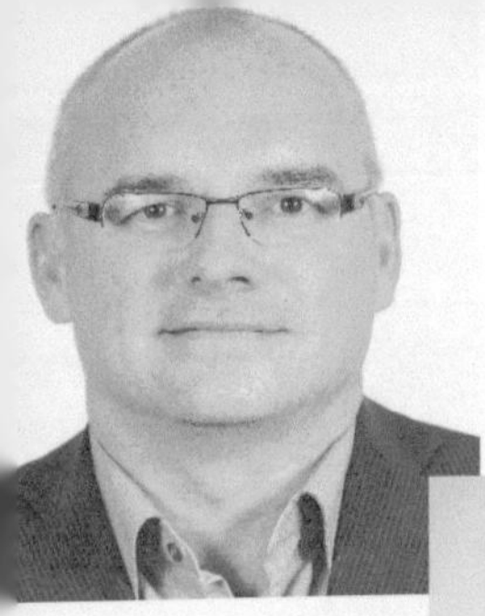
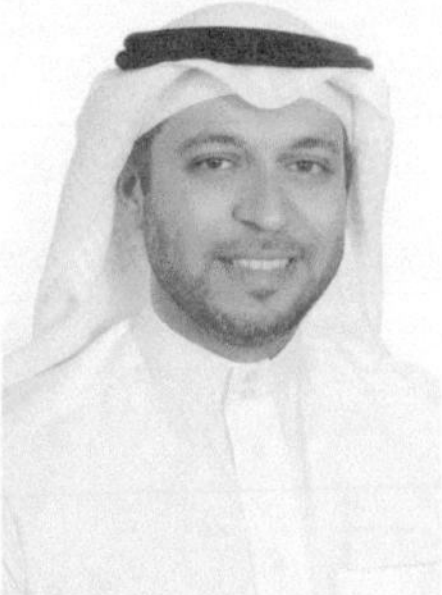
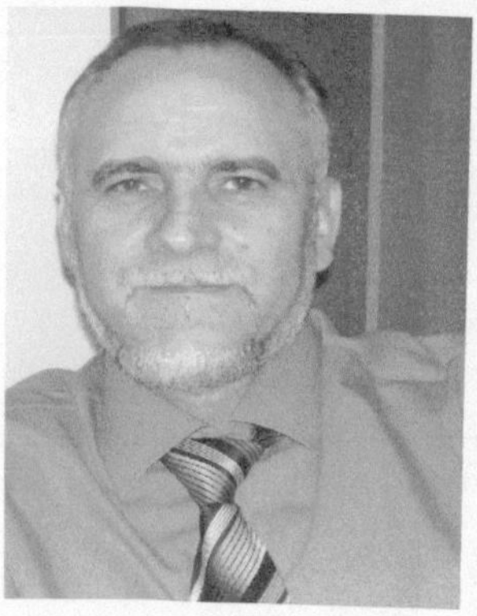
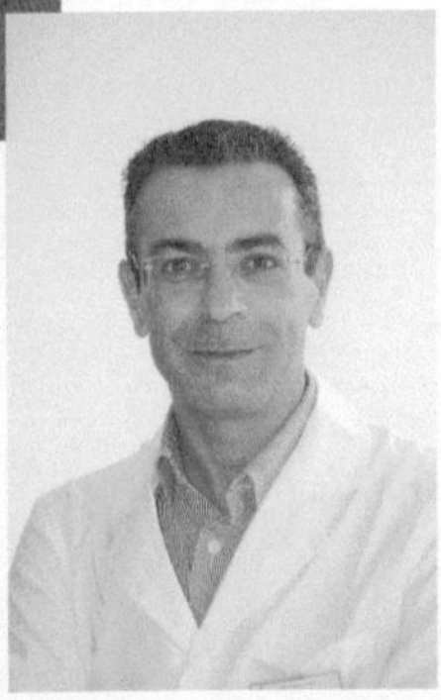
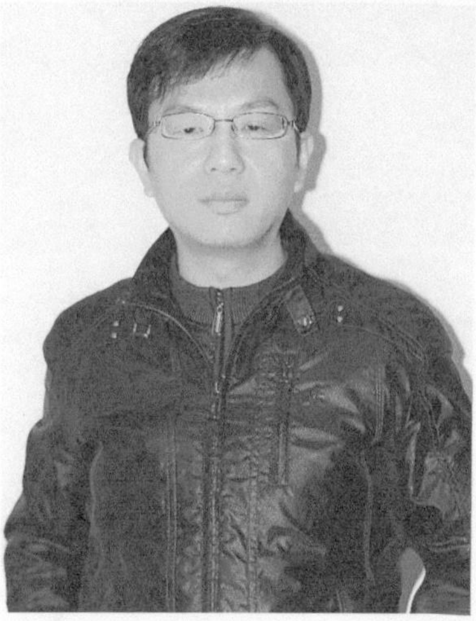
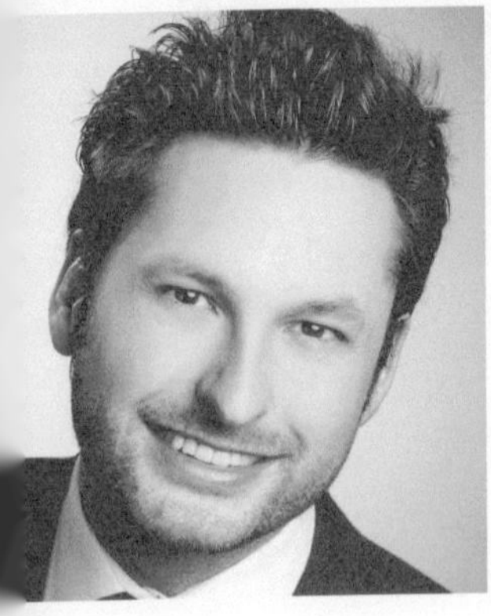
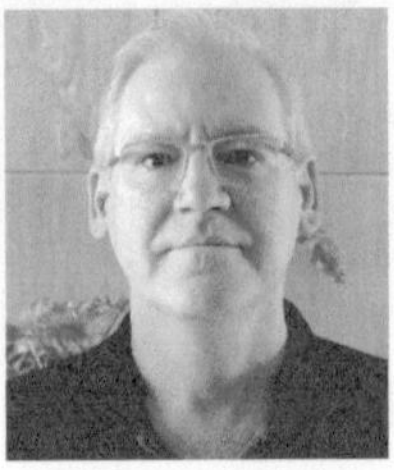

IntechOpen

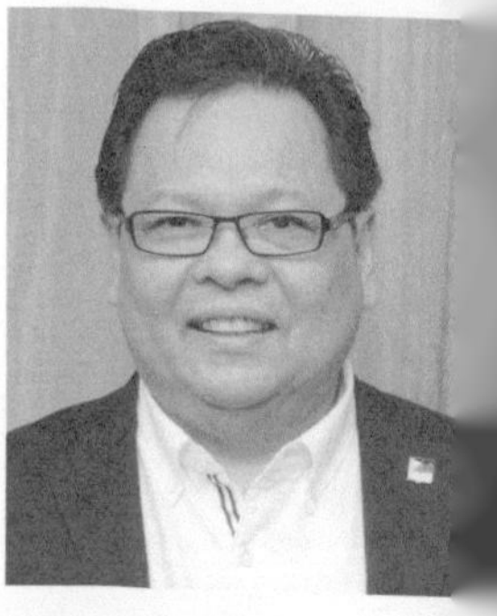
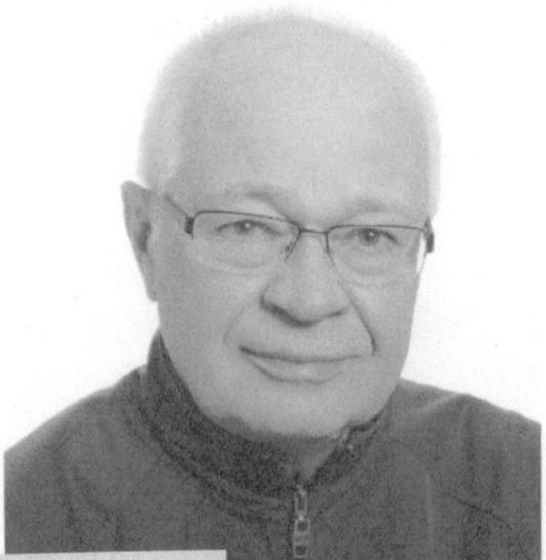
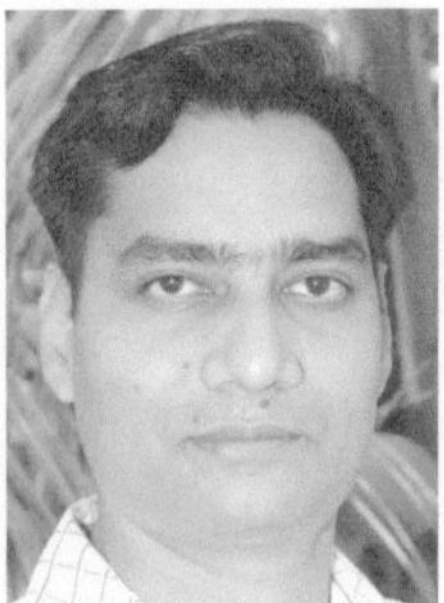
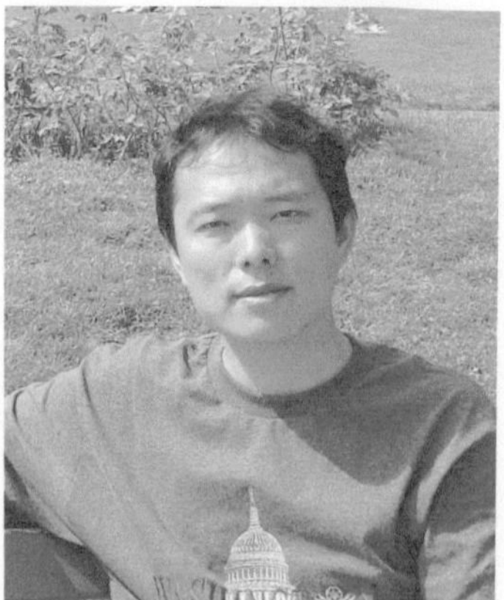
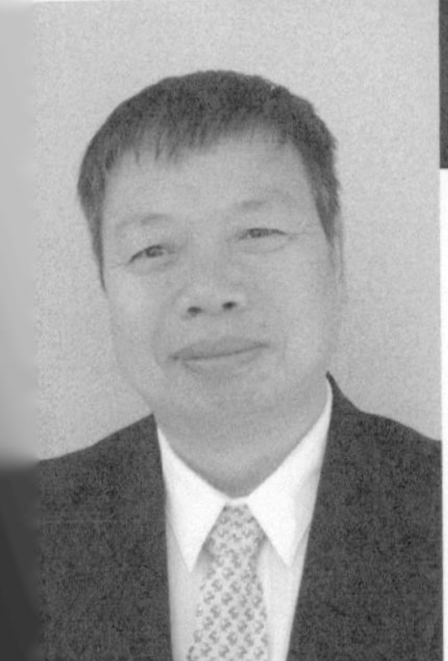
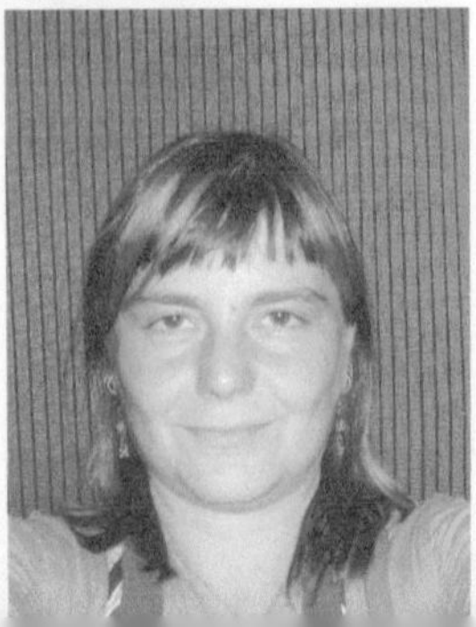

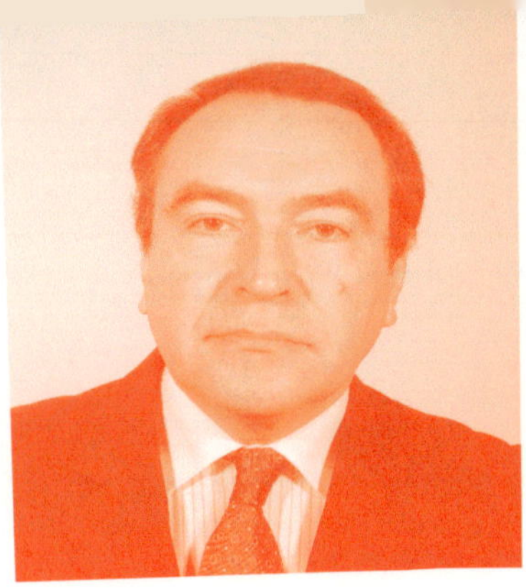
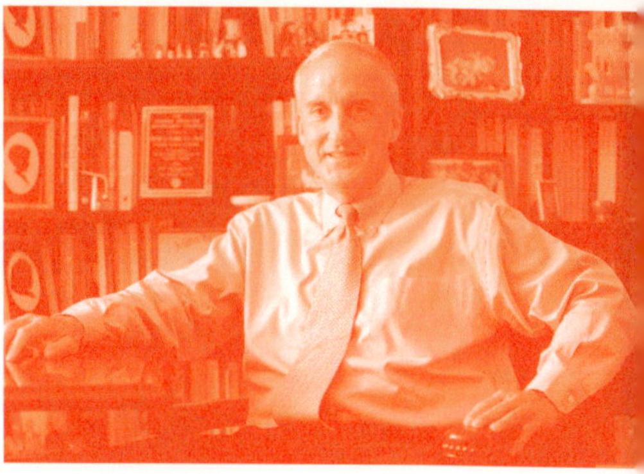
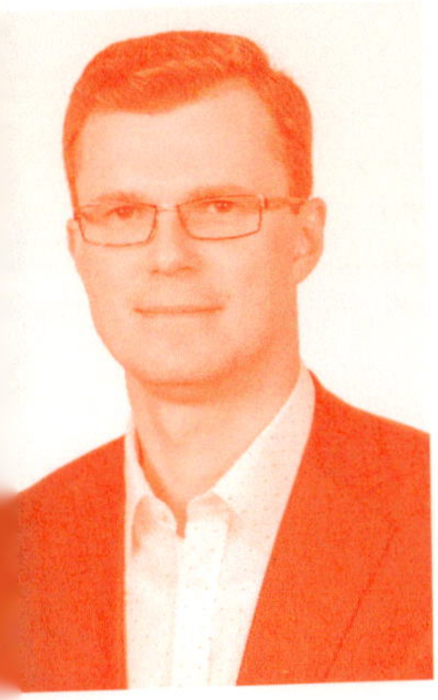
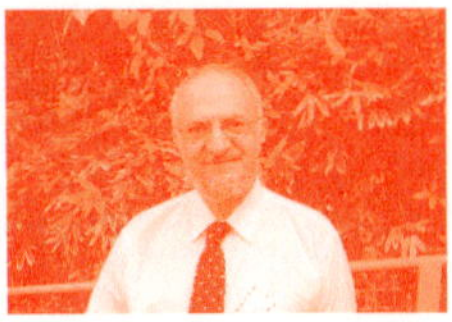
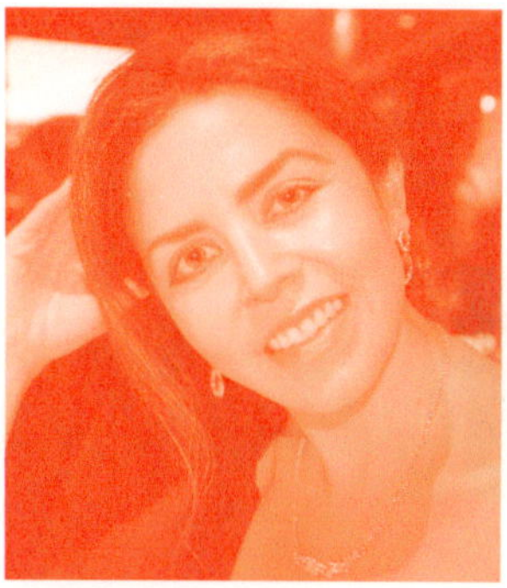

Supporting open minds since 2005

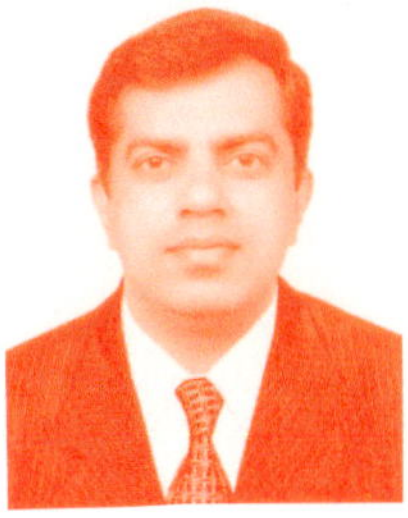
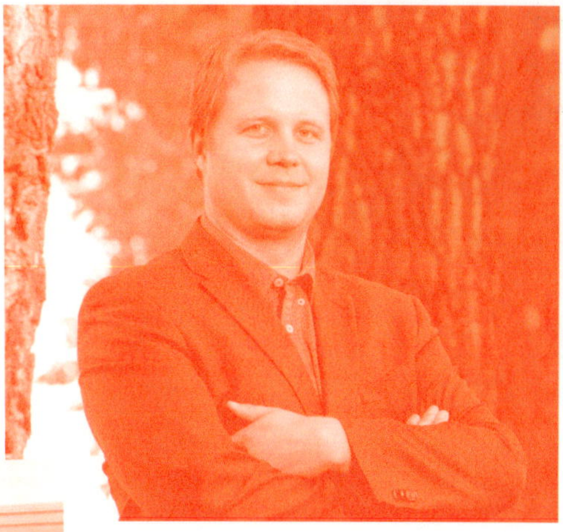
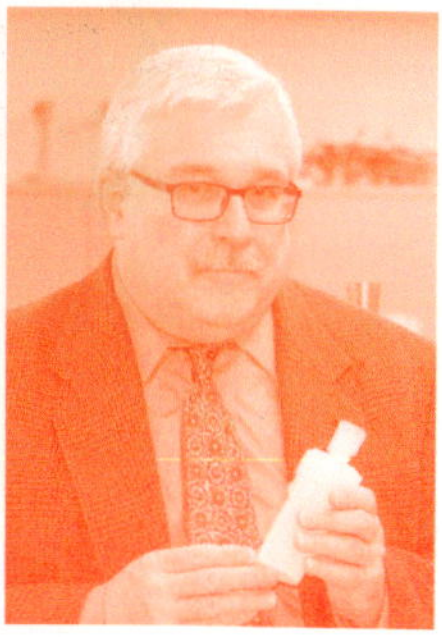
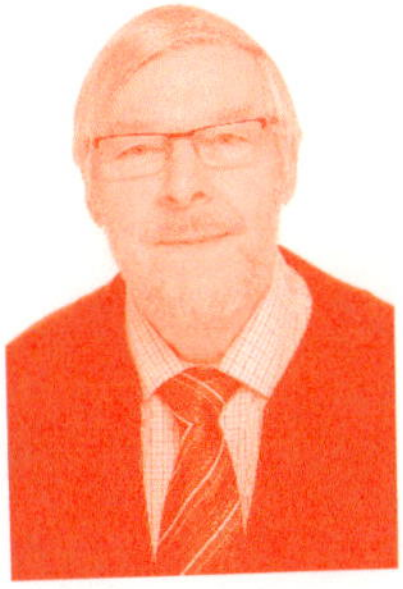
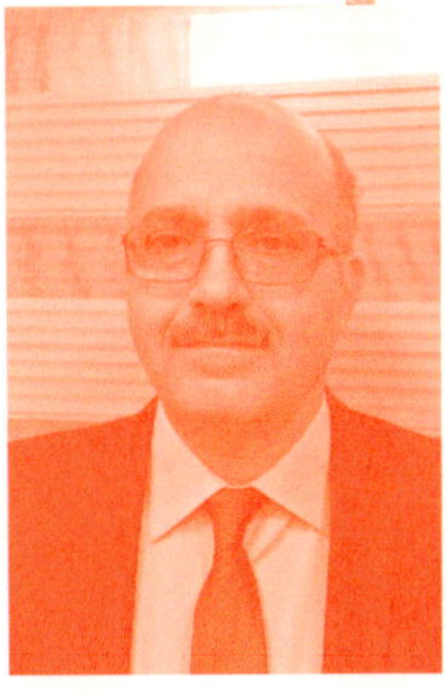
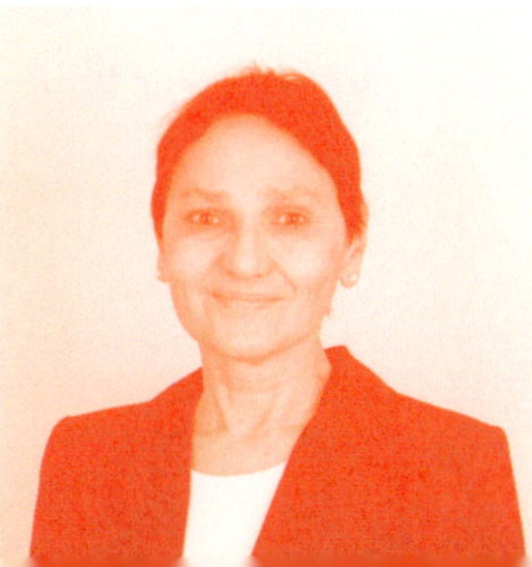
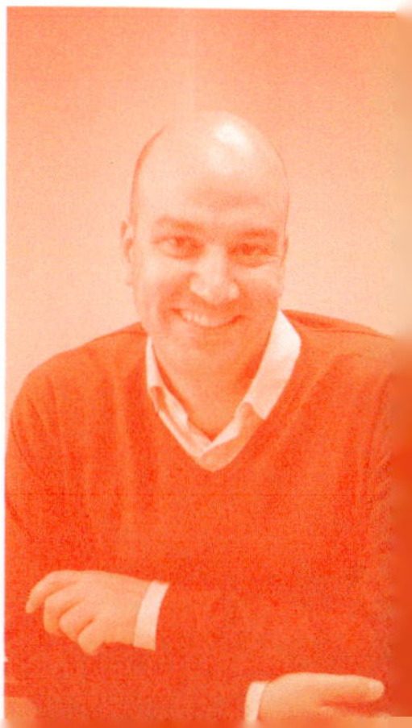

Thymus
http://dx.doi.org/10.5772/intechopen.73777
Edited by Nima Rezaei

Contributors
Dragoş Cătălin Jianu, Silviana Nina Jianu, Claudia Birsan, Rachel Thomas, Dong-Ming Su, Sarai Belchi-Navarro, Ana-Belen Sabater-Jara, María Pina Funes, Maria A. Pedreño, Ali Kouhi, Saeed Sohrabpour, Krisztian Kvell, Ildikó Bódi, Krisztina H.-Minkó, Zsolt Prodán, Imre Oláh, Robin Cornelissen, Arbab Sikandar, Shahzaib Shahzaib, Naeem Ullah, Teresa Fortoul, Martha Ustarroz-Cano, Nelly López-Valdez, Isabel García-Peláez, Marisol Lopea-Angel, Nima Rezaei, Amene Saghazadeh

First published in London, United Kingdom, 2020 by IntechOpen
IntechOpen is the global imprint of INTECHOPEN LIMITED, registered in England and Wales, registration number: 11086078, 7th floor, 10 Lower Thames Street, London, EC3R 6AF, United Kingdom
Printed in Croatia

British Library Cataloguing-in-Publication Data
A catalogue record for this book is available from the British Library

Additional hard and PDF copies can be obtained from orders@intechopen.com

Thymus
Edited by Nima Rezaei
p. cm.
Print ISBN 978-1-78985-133-5
Online ISBN 978-1-78985-134-2
eBook (PDF) ISBN 978-1-83968-559-0

Meet the editor

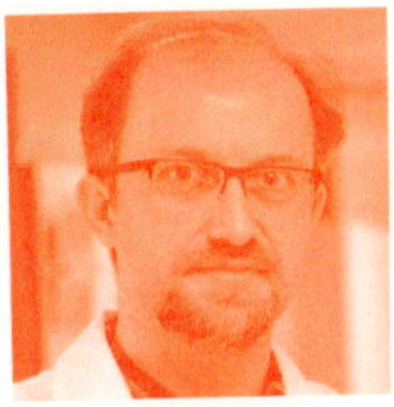

Professor Nima Rezaei obtained an MD from Tehran University of Medical Sciences, and an MSc in Molecular and Genetic Medicine and PhD in Clinical Immunology and Human Genetics from the University of Sheffield, UK. Dr. Rezai also spent a short-term fellowship in Pediatric Clinical Immunology and Bone Marrow Transplantation at the Newcastle General Hospital. He is now Full Professor of Immunology and Vice Dean of International Affairs, School of Medicine, Tehran University of Medical Sciences, and the co-founder and Deputy President of the Research Center for Immunodeficiencies. He is also the founding president of the Universal Scientific Education and Research Network (USERN). Prof. Rezaei has already been the director of more than 50 research projects and has designed and participated in several international collaborative projects. He is an editorial assistant or board member for more than 30 international journals. He has edited more than 10 international books, has presented more than 400 lectures/posters in congresses/meetings, and has published more than 700 articles in international scientific journals.

Contents

Preface

As an immunologist, I am used to emphasizing the importance of the thymus gland. This gland is extremely important in that it plays a vital role in the training and development of T cells.

This book opens with a brief introduction to the thymus, including its development and functions. Subsequent chapters examine a range of conditions – including environmental pollution, congenital anomalies, autoimmune diseases, and malignancies – that threaten the function and development of this gland. The volume also considers that the thymus undergoes aging and examines dietary supplementation as a way to sustain its life.

Nima Rezaei, M.D., Ph.D.
Research Center for Immunodeficiencies,
Children's Medical Center,
Tehran University of Medical Sciences,
Tehran, Iran

Network of Immunity in Infection,
Malignancy and Autoimmunity (NIIMA),
Universal Scientific Education and Research Network (USERN),
Tehran, Iran

Chapter 1

Introductory Chapter: Thymus - The Central Self-Tolerance System

Amene Saghazadeh and Nima Rezaei

1. Where, when, and why of the thymus

The pharynx is regarded as a part of the digestive system. It is, however, attached to the respiratory system and, thus, is referred to as the conducting zone of the respiratory system as well. The pharyngeal apparatus groups together five pharyngeal arches, four pharyngeal pouches, four pharyngeal clefts, and pharyngeal membranes that occur during 4–5 weeks of human development [1]. Within the developmental context, the thymus is closely related to parathyroid glands [2] since both are derived from the endodermal-lined pharyngeal pouches—the thymus develops from the ventral portion of pouch 3, and the inferior and superior parathyroid glands arise from the dorsal portions of pouches 3 and 4, respectively.

Late in the 4th week, the primordia of the thymus begin to form but remain attached to that of the inferior parathyroid glands for a time [3]. By the 7th week, they migrate to the position where they should reside and be functional—the thymus is located midline in the upper chest just behind the sternum between the lungs and above the heart, and the inferior parathyroid glands descend along the inferior border of the thyroid. However, it takes about 12 weeks to form the definitive structure of the thymus, a bilobed organ that is covered by a mesenchymal capsule and is composed of two internal layers: the cortex and the medulla. The cortex is the outer layer of the thymus in which cortical thymic epithelial cells (cTECs) are found. The medulla is located in the center of the thymus. It is where medullary thymic epithelial cells (mTECs) and Hassall's (thymic) corpuscles are present.

The thymus is seen as of high value, due to its functions as a part of the neuroendocrine system in addition to its actions to provide a primary lymphoid microenvironment that efficiently carries T cell differentiation and selection. The first evidence that the thymus can have immune and endocrine functions was provided from athymic nude animals and/or animals undergoing thymectomy showing impairments in their cell-mediated immunity, growth pattern, and puberty and developing organ-specific autoimmune diseases. These impairments were consistent with their relative reduction in levels of thyroxin, testosterone, progesterone, and 17-β-estradiol, whereas corticosterone levels were elevated. Of particular note was that the passive transfer of lymphocytes and thymus implantation at birth were effective in transferring cell-mediated immunity to nude mice [4]. The endocrine defects could be, in part, healed by thymus implantation at birth as well but remain stable following passive transfer of lymphoid cells [4].

IntechOpen

2. How does the thymus teach T lymphocytes self-tolerance?

2.1 Immunological tolerance

To keep the body healthy, the immune system is expected to entail invading pathogens while avoiding reactivity to self-tissues. This so-called immunological tolerance engages both central and peripheral modes of action (for review, see [5]).

2.1.1 Central tolerance

It is referred to immature B and T cells when they are present in the primary lymphoid organs—B cells in the bone marrow and T cells in the thymus. Mechanisms of central tolerance are, for example, clonal deletion and elimination of self-reactive cells.

2.1.2 Peripheral tolerance

This one is for mature B and T cells as detached from the primary lymphoid organs into the bloodstream, lymph, and secondary lymphoid organs such as spleen and lymph nodes. There are various mechanisms that can promote tolerance in the periphery, including clonal deletion, clonal anergy, clonal ignorance, deviation, helplessness, and suppression.

2.2 Thymopoiesis: the result of cross-talk between thymic stromal cells and precursor T cells

T cell progenitors that lack both CD4 and CD8 receptors are termed as double-negative (DN) cells. These cells separate from the bone marrow, enter the thymus through the large venules located at the corticomedullary junction (CMJ), and settle into the cortex of the thymus. In the thymic cortex, the rearrangement at T cell receptor (TCR) α and β genes makes the cells turn into double-positive (DP) stage, when cells express both CD4 and CD8. Then, a positive selection process directs DP cells into either CD4+ or CD8+ T cells depending on their affinity for either major histocompatibility complex (MHC) protein class II or I, respectively. The thymus selects single-positive (SP) immunocompetent T cells to export them out of the thymus. In the periphery, these naïve self-restricted T cells eventually home to secondary lymphoid organs. To bear the name of its creators, i.e., thymocytes, this process of manufacturing mature functional T cells is generally recognized as thymopoiesis.

2.3 Thymic mechanisms of central self-tolerance

2.3.1 Positive selection takes place in the thymic cortex

The positive selection is defined as a process through which SP T cells expressing either CD4 or CD8 are selected. The thymic cortex carries gene rearrangements that make precursor T cells co-express CD4 and CD8. These DP T cells are then engaged by a ligand bound to an MHC class II or I molecule that is present on cTECs and will be differentiated into SP T cells that express either CD4 or CD8, correspondingly [6].

2.3.2 Negative selection takes place in the thymic medulla

The negative selection is simply a process by which autoreactive T cells are removed. After positive selection is done, the transfer of SP T cells from the cortex to the medulla occurs. The expression of chemokine receptor CCR7 by T cells is essential to the transfer process—since antigen-presenting cells (APCs) including mTECs and dendritic cells in the medulla express CCR7 ligands, e.g., CCL19 and CCL21. In this manner, SP T cells can engage in interaction with medullary APCs that present a variety of tissue-restricted antigens (TRAs). Medullary APCs are responsible for finding autoreactive T cells that recognize self-antigen—MHC complexes and their removal. Such selection would permit SP T cells that are not reactive to self to shift from the thymus to the periphery [6].

2.3.3 Agonist selection takes place in the thymic medulla

The agonist selection is also undertaken by the thymic medulla to allow a portion of autoreactive CD4+ T cells to differentiate into regulatory T (Treg) cells that express forkhead box P3 (Foxp3). These regulatory T cells that are derived from the thymus are referred to as tTreg cells and move from the thymus to the peripheral tissues. They constitute the majority of all Treg cells and play the central role in immune tolerance. So, the thymus must be precisely effective in the generation of Treg cells. If this could not be achieved, then we see the process of autoimmunity. However, there are Treg cells derived from peripheral tissues referred to as pTreg cells. This type of Treg cells is especially accumulated at sites of inflammation and consequently regulates inflammatory responses [6].

3. If peace is in the hands of the thymus, then what would happen if that does not work?

The thymus-mediated effects including the production of neuropeptides and also development of T cell repertoire are what may be called the function of the pacemaker [7]. However, the thymus is vulnerable to be exposed to both acute and chronic injuries. A variety of pathological conditions that range from infections and immunodeficiency to inflammatory and autoimmune disorders and tumors may cause the thymus to turn into malfunctioning or functionless. In a broader sense, the thymus undergoes physiological changes that occur with age and during pregnancy. Below is to represent dysregulation of immune homeostasis as the inevitable consequence of a failure in central self-tolerance system, i.e., the thymus.

3.1 The effects of thymic infection on thymopoiesis

3.1.1 The thymus gets sick

The thymus is not immune-privileged, but rather invading pathogens can adversely affect its structure and/or function, thymopoiesis, through indirect (systemic) and direct (local) ways. Pathogens that are able to penetrate into the different thymic location(s), e.g., cortex, CMJ, or medulla, and thereby directly infect thymic cells, include a number of viruses (human immunodeficiency virus, *Simian immunodeficiency virus*, influenza virus, lymphocytic choriomeningitis virus, *Murine leukemia virus*, mouse hepatitis virus, human cytomegalovirus, measles virus, coxsackievirus, Epstein-Barr virus, Junin virus, and poliovirus), bacteria (*Mycobacterium avium*, *Mycobacterium tuberculosis*, *Francisella tularensis*, and *Salmonella enterica*), fungi (*Paracoccidioides brasiliensis* and *Cryptococcus neoformans*), and parasites (*Trypanosoma cruzi*, *Plasmodium berghei*, and *Toxoplasma gondii*). In addition, pathogens can act indirectly by altering the systemic expression of glucocorticoids, cytokines, chemokines, and antigens. Then, these soluble factors can reach the village of the thymus and readily result in changes of its microenvironment [8].

Without regard to the nature of its invading pathogens, the infected thymus may encounter atrophy and architectural changes. The infected thymus is consequently liable to induce apoptosis, pathogen-specific immune responses, T cells that are tolerant to pathogens, and self-reactive T cells [8].

3.1.2 The thymus can cope with infection

Less is understood for mechanisms of thymic escape from infection and/or survival after being infected. However, it is suggested that the thymus may be affected by seeding of cells from other peripheral sites of infection. Therefore, elimination of infection from other peripheral sites might help in the prevention of seeding and development of infection in the thymus. When it gets infected, there is evidence on the presence of antigen-specific CD4+ or CD8+ T cells of other peripheral organs. This would imply that the thymus might in time profit from responses mediated by effector T cells that recirculate between peripheral tissues [8].

3.2 The role of thymic involution in the aging immune system

3.2.1 The thymus gets old

Older individuals have higher rates of diseases, e.g., infections, malignancies, and autoimmune diseases, demonstrate lower responsiveness to vaccines, and are less capable of immune restoration following chemotherapy, radiotherapy, and infections. This is plainly a reflection of the aging immune system, referred to as immune senescence, related to increased mortality and morbidity in the aged population. The immune cells mostly affected by aging are naïve T cells [9]. Yet the number of memory cells is proportionally increased. The process of T cell-mediated immunity becoming deteriorated gradually occurs, and both extrinsic and intrinsic factors may play a role [10].

Rather than being influenced by bone marrow aging, age-related deterioration of T cell-mediated immunity is influenced by the thymic involution. Both are, however, seated to serve as co-directors of this process. When the thymus undergoes aging, its architecture does not remain well defined. Cellular changes associated with thymic involution include reduction in the number of thymic epithelial cells and thymocytes in contrast to an increase in perivascular spaces and adipose tissue. Aging will affect the bone marrow in parallel to the thymus, making the quantity and quality of progenitor T cells that migrate from the bone marrow to the thymus go down. When "progenitor T cells" are not inputted to the "thymus" machine, then the output "naïve T cells" would not be logic anymore. In this manner, aging causes a decline in naïve T cells exported from the thymus to the periphery, and consequently memory T cells will predominate in the periphery.

3.2.2 The thymus has the ability to sustain life

Thymic involution is characterized by a continuous flow from the first year of life that gets pronounced at puberty and during pregnancy. After puberty, the thymus gradually decreases in size, weight, and cellularity as we age, and by the seventh decade of life, the thymic epithelial space drops to less than 10 percent of total tissue. This fact that the thymus feels old when the levels of sex steroids and hormones rise [9] provides, as a result, a role for sex steroids in the aging of the thymus. It also will open our eyes to see sex steroid ablation as a potential means of regenerating the thymus and consequently reversing immune senescence. There is reasonable evidence to believe that the prevention and/or reversal of thymic function associated with aging is possible with sex steroid ablation using surgical and pharmaceutical approaches [11].

Thymopoiesis is an active complex process. Growth-stimulating factors, such as hematopoietic cytokines (interleukin-1, interleukin-3, interleukin-6, interleukin-7, interleukin-21, and interleukin-22, stem cell factor, and FMS-like tyrosine kinase 3 ligand), growth factors (transforming growth factor beta, oncostatin M, keratinocyte growth factor, bone morphogenetic protein 4, leukemia inhibitory factor), and hormones (growth hormone, insulin growth factor 1, and ghrelin), are, thus, needed to facilitate the cooperation between the two parties, i.e., thymocytes and T cells, involved in thymopoiesis. There are reports that the age-associated defects in the immune function and/or structure of the thymus could be returned by the administration of these factors (for review, see [11–13]). In particular, interleukin-21 has provided the most interesting results, as explained in preclinical studies [12].

Similarly, bioengineering thymus organoids [14], thymus transplantation, and cell-based therapies have been effective in immune reconstitution and establishing immune tolerance to allografts.

Author details

Amene Saghazadeh[1,2] and Nima Rezaei[1,3,4*]

1 Research Center for Immunodeficiencies, Children's Medical Center, Tehran University of Medical Sciences (TUMS), Tehran, Iran

2 Systematic Review and Meta-analysis Expert Group (SRMEG), Universal Scientific Education and Research Network (USERN), Tehran, Iran

3 Department of Immunology, School of Medicine, Tehran University of Medical Sciences (TUMS), Tehran, Iran

4 Network of Immunity in Infection, Malignancy and Autoimmunity (NIIMA), Universal Scientific Education and Research Network (USERN), Tehran, Iran

*Address all correspondence to: rezaei_nima@yahoo.com

References

[1] Sadler TW. Langman's Medical Embryology. Philadelphia Pa London: Lippincott Williams & Wilkins; 2011

[2] Gordon J, Manley NR. Mechanisms of thymus organogenesis and morphogenesis. Development. 2011;**138**(18):3865-3878

[3] Larsen WJ. Human Embryology. Churchill Livingstone; 2001. Available from: https://www.elsevier.com/books/larsens-human-embryology/schoenwolf/978-1-4557-0684-6

[4] Pierpaoli W, Besedovsky HO. Role of the thymus in programming of neuroendocrine functions. Clinical and Experimental Immunology. 1975;**20**(2):323

[5] Mathis D, Benoist C. Back to central tolerance. Immunity. 2004;**20**(5):509-516

[6] Takaba H, Takayanagi H. The mechanisms of T cell selection in the thymus. Trends in Immunology. 2017;**38**(11):805-816

[7] Csaba G. The immunoendocrine thymus as a pacemaker of lifespan. Acta Microbiologica et Immunologica Hungarica. 2016;**63**(2):139-158

[8] Nunes-Alves C et al. Tolerance has its limits: How the thymus copes with infection. Trends in Immunology. 2013;**34**(10):502-510

[9] Calder AE et al. Thymic involution: Where endocrinology meets immunology. Neuroimmunomodulation. 2011;**18**(5):281-289

[10] Palmer D. The effect of age on thymic function. Frontiers in Immunology. 2013;**4**:316

[11] Ventevogel MS, Sempowski GD. Thymic rejuvenation and aging. Current Opinion in Immunology. 2013;**25**(4):516-522

[12] El-Kadiry AE-H, Rafei M. Restoring thymic function: Then and now. Cytokine. 2019;**120**:202-209

[13] Chaudhry MS et al. Thymus: The next (re)generation. Immunological Reviews. 2016;**271**(1):56-71

[14] Fan Y et al. Bioengineering thymus organoids to restore thymic function and induce donor-specific immune tolerance to allografts. Molecular Therapy. 2015;**23**(7):1262-1277

Chapter 2

Compartmentalization of Human Thymic Medulla: Facts and Hypotheses

Ildiko Bodi, Krisztina H.-Minko, Zsolt Prodan and Imre Olah

Abstract

The thymus function was discovered in the middle of the last century. The role of the thymus in the adaptive immune system facilitated its histological and experimental studies. Before the role of the thymus was discovered, the thymus was called as a gland on the basis of lobulation; even some histological textbook listed it up among the endocrine glands. In addition to the cortex and medulla, the immunohistochemical studies revealed a further compartmentalization in the thymic medulla, which is related to the epithelium-free areas (EFA) and keratin-positive network (KPN). The two medullary compartments have different cellularity that determines their role. This chapter would concentrate on the medullary compartmentalization and their cellularity. Furthermore, this chapter discusses the relationship of thymic septae with the perivascular space, the vascular embedding and thymic dendritic cells.

Keywords: medulla, epithelium-free area, keratin-positive network, dendritic cells

1. Introduction

In the histological textbooks, the main morphological landmarks of the thymus are (1) the lobulation—like the glands; (2) the darkly and lightly stained cortex and medulla, respectively; and (3) the Hassall's bodies. The relatively simple structure of the thymus did not help to "decode" the enigmatic thymic function until the middle of the last century. The three morphological landmarks may be supplemented by the keratin-negative area (KNA) [1, 2] or "epithelium-free area" (EFA) [3–6]. EFA can be found in both the cortex and medulla [6–8]. In the cortex, the EFA is a nest of double-positive (CD4+, CD8+) T lymphocytes [4] and various macrophages [7]. Others suggest that the cortical EFA is a pathological phenomenon [3, 6].

If the KNA/EFA is a permanent compartment of the human thymic medulla, then it should be added to the general histological features of the thymus of the warm-blooded vertebrates.

2. Relationship between perivascular space (PVS) and keratin-negative and/or epithelium-free areas

In the medulla, the perivascular space (PVS) [7, 9–12]—that is, the dilated primary septum (PS)—carries the blood vessels, which locate "outside" the basal lamina of the thymus [1, 2, 12, 13], but Foxn-1, which is a thymic epithelial cell-specific

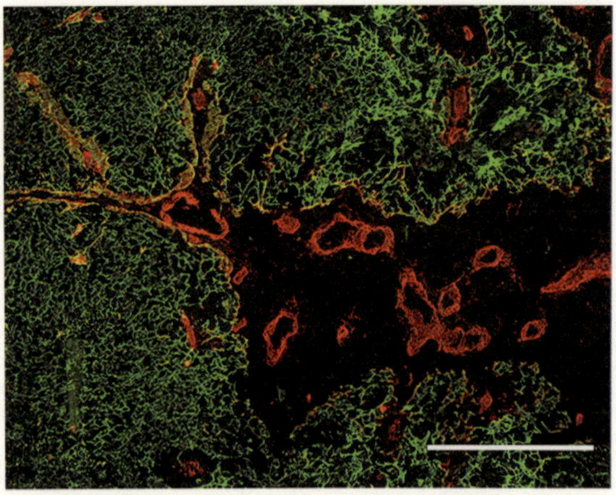

Figure 1.
Double staining of chicken thymus: cytokeratin (green) and laminin (red). At the PS, the laminin shows a continuous basal lamina, which becomes discontinuous in the EFA. The KNA/PVS receives the blood vessels.

transcription factor [14], regulates thymic vascularization [15]. At the cortico-medullary junction, PS merges to the PVS of the medulla [9, 10]. A continuous basal lamina covers the thymic parenchyma toward the capsule and PS, and it becomes discontinuous at the end of the PS (**Figure 1**) [2, 7] where it turns to be the PVS or KNA/EFA. In the thymic medulla, the lack of blood-thymus barrier [16] may be explained by the discontinuity of the basal lamina on the border of the KNA/EFA [2]. The discontinuity of the basal lamina suggests that the microenvironment of the KNA/EFA and PVS is identical. Silver impregnation shows that both the PS and the KNA/EFA consist of reticular connective tissue [2, 9, 17] and have common extracellular matrix [11]. Secondary septae appear after formation of the cortex and medulla, and they are just small invaginations of the capsule and usually do not reach the medulla and do not receive blood vessels. The medullary EFA occupies about one-fifth of the rat thymus [18]. In chicken our morphometric studies confirm the considerable size of the KNA, that is, close to 50% of the medulla [2]. The border of the keratin-positive network (KPN) and KNA is an epithelial-mesenchymal border that could be the functional cortico-medullary (CM) border of the thymus [2]. The KPN-KNA/EFA border is supported by cellular background, unlike the hematoxylin-eosin-stained, classical CM border, which is based only on lymphocyte density and subsequently stainability. The mesenchymal tissue of the PVS develops from neural crest cells [19–22]. The PVS is a transit zone of migratory cells between the thymus and circulation [12, 23].

Anti-cytokeratin immunostaining identifies the KPN and KNA/EFA in both embryonic and postembryonic chicken thymuses. In an 11-day-old chicken embryo, the thymic epithelial anlage shows a starfish-shaped form (**Figure 2**). Between the 5–6 secondary epithelial cords, the unstained PS(s) consist of mesenchyme. During the next two ED (11 and 13), the cortical epithelial cells rapidly proliferate resulting in enlarged thymic rudiment (**Figure 3**) which is colonized by hematopoietic cells. In 11-ED-old birds, the wide PS became narrow, and the bottom of the PS is involved into the medulla as the KNA/EFA.

The PS is going on as the KNA/EFA, and both regions consist of reticular connective tissue stained with silver impregnation [2, 6, 17, 24]. Mesenchymal markers desmin and ER-TR7 [6, 25] revealed specific staining in the capsule, septae, and medullary PVS. In the PVS, the neural crest cells differentiate into smooth muscle cells of thymic blood vessels and pericytes of thymic capillaries [21]. These histological findings suggest the common origin of the PS and KNA/EFA: namely, the KNA/EFA develops from the cranial neural crest cells [19, 21, 26].

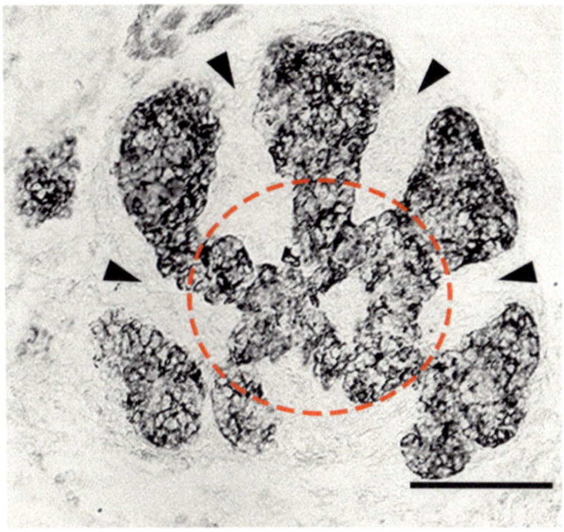

Figure 2.
11 ED chicken thymus: anti-cytokeratin. The starfish-shaped epithelial thymic anlage shows the branching of the primary epithelial cord to 5–6 secondary cords. The dashed circle outlines the future medulla.

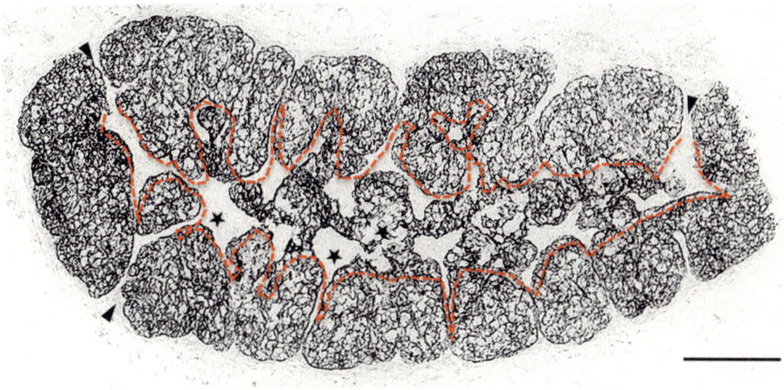

Figure 3.
13 ED chicken thymus: the rapid proliferation of epithelial cells enlarged the thymic cortical epithelium. The bottom of the PS (arrowhead) dilates and becomes the KNA/EFA of medulla (star).

3. Keratin-negative area/epithelium-free area

Mesenchymal cells and fibroblasts express vimentin intermediate filament. Cortical thymocytes and epithelial cells are vimentin negative (**Figure 4**), but thymic medulla shows homogenous staining pattern, indicating that keratin-positive and keratin-negative compartments cannot be distinguished (**Figure 5**). The homogenous vimentin staining of the medulla may indicate that the medullary epithelial cells express vimentin intermediate filament. Hassall's bodies are vimentin negative (**Figure 5**), like cortical epithelial cells. In the majority of vimentin-positive cells, the immunoreaction appears in the periphery of the cell cytoplasm. The nature of the medullary vimentin-positive cells is not clear, because vimentin can colocalize with other intermediate filaments, like neurofilament, cytokeratin, and desmin; therefore the anti-vimentin immunostaining used for identification of mesenchymal cells is limited [25]. Blood vessels and dendritic cells are the most significant structures of the KNA/EFA. Anti-von Willebrand factor identifies endothelial cells (**Figure 6**). Transmission electron microscopy shows the organelle-rich cytoplasm of the interdigitating dendritic cell (IDC) (**Figure 7**). The IDC is located in close association with the blood vessels [2].

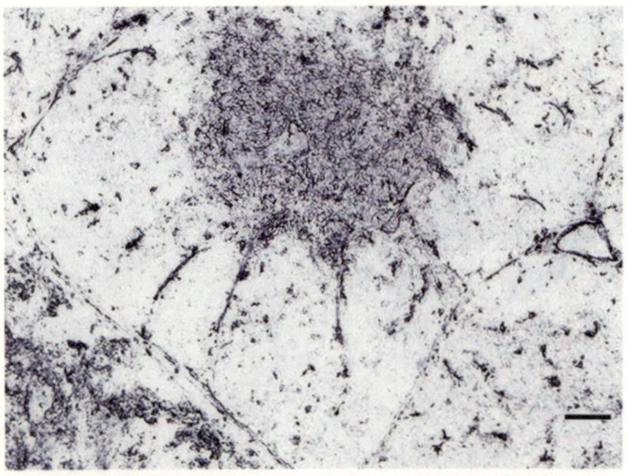

Figure 4.
Anti-vimentin antibody outlines the capsule and PS. The cortical epithelial cells and T cells are negative, while all medullary cells express vimentin. C, cortex; M, medulla.

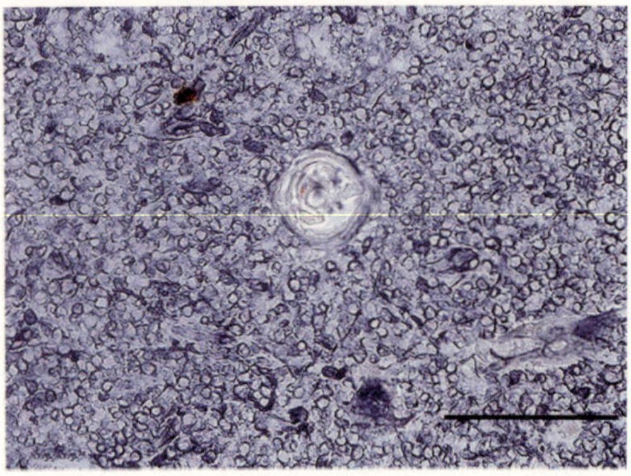

Figure 5.
Higher magnification of anti-vimentin-stained thymic medulla. The round-shaped Hassall's body is negative, while the medullary cells show a round-shaped-positive reaction.

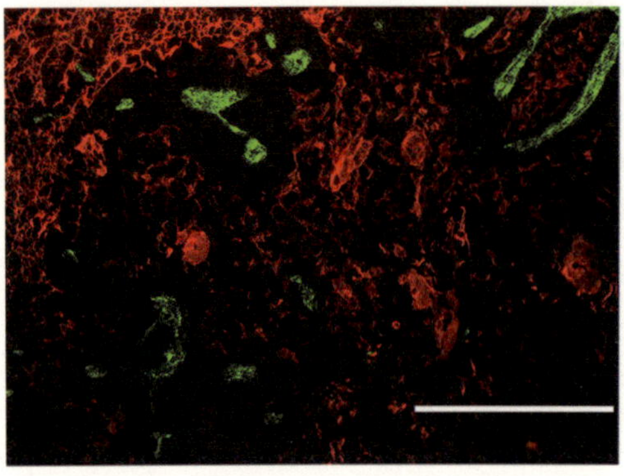

Figure 6.
Double staining: cytokeratin (red) and von Willebrand factor (green). Blood vessels exclusively locate in the KNA/EFA.

As mentioned above, the PVS consists of mesenchymal cells of neural crest origin; therefore, the supporting tissue of the KNA/EFA is also mesenchyme. The thickness of the PVS is used to be in one or two cell layers, but in chicken thymus, the morphometric studies show that the ratio between keratin-positive and keratin-negative fields is close to one to one [2]. Considerable size of the KNA/EFA

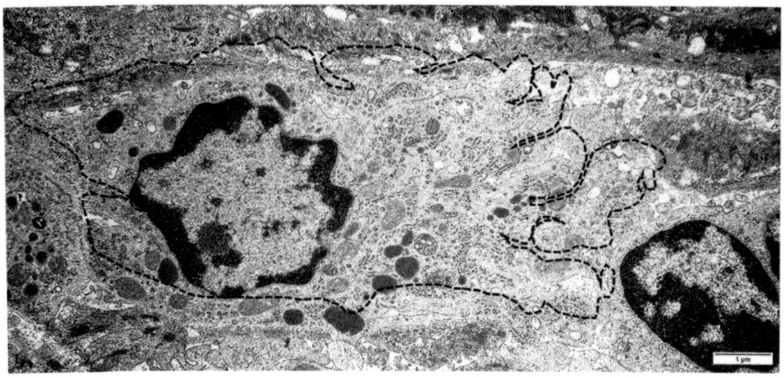

Figure 7.
Transmission electron micrograph of a thymic dendritic cell. The cell membrane is outlined. The cytoplasm is rich in organelles and electron-dense granules.

(**Figure 6**) suggests that its functional significance must be more than a passive transit zone for cell migration between circulation and the thymus [4, 10–12]. Thymic IDC [9] is located in the KNA/EFA [2] and contributes to T-cell selection. In nonobese mouse, autoimmune type I diabetes develops, resulting in abnormal distribution of epithelial cells and consequently giant PVS [11, 17]. After cyclosporin A (CyA) treatment of the rats, the thymic medulla disappeared, and 2 weeks after CyA treatment, the recovery of the medulla took place, but the "holes" were epithelial cell-free [5]. The occurrence and size of the KNA/EFA may be varied from species to species [2] even among the strains of rats [3]. In the CM region of BB rat thymus, the EFA has been reported, but this KNA/EFA is not as complete as in man. In the thymic medulla, the frequency of the KNA/EFA alters by age: in young Wistar rats, the occurrence of the KNA/EFA is higher than in old animals [7]. These changes may be related to acute [5] and/or physiological thymic involution.

The thymic stromal elements develop from the endodermal epithelium and neural crest mesenchyme. Hematopoietic cells colonize the epithelial-mesenchymal anlage. In chicken embryo the KNA/EFA appears when the medulla and cortex differentiate; therefore the epithelial-mesenchymal transition [6] would create a "second" mesenchyme, besides the mesenchyme of cranial neural crest origin. Therefore, in the thymus the epithelial-mesenchymal transition may be redundant.

It was difficult to identify large epithelium-free areas by transmission electron microscopy, and Foxn-1 thymic epithelial cell-specific transcription factor showed

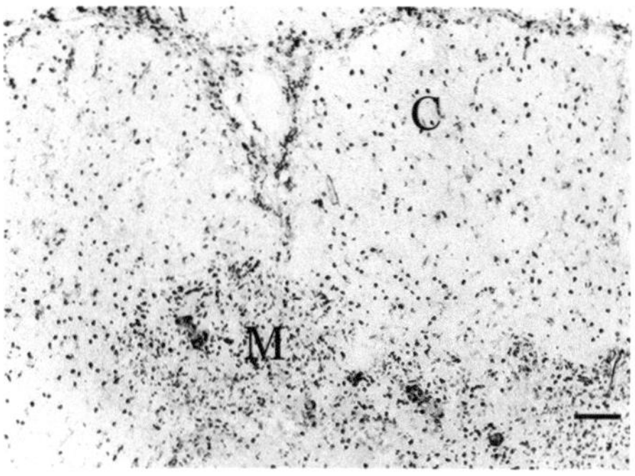

Figure 8.
Thymus 5. Age 16 months: Foxn-1 antibody recognizes epithelial nuclei over the entire thymus. Density of Foxn-1-positive cells is higher in the medulla (M) than in the cortex (C). The Foxn-1-positive knots are possibly Hassall's bodies.

positive cells in the KNA/EFA (**Figure 8**). Foxn-1 expression in the medullary KNA/EFA is a puzzle. In early embryogenesis, Foxn-1 expresses in several mesenchymal and epithelial cells [27]; therefore one of the possibilities for solving the puzzle is that Foxn-1 is maintained in the KNA/EFA after thymus development. The other possibility is that the thymic epithelial cells induce Foxn-1 expression in mesenchymal cells of cranial neural crest origin [28]. Removal of perithymic mesenchyme at ED12 or culture of purified ED14 epithelial cells alone resulted in a threefold reduction in the bromodeoxyuridine incorporation by keratin-positive cells. Proliferation of thymic epithelial cells in the early thymus is regulated by signals from mesenchyme [29]. These mesenchymal cells produce fibroblast growth factors 7 and 10, which stimulate epithelial cell proliferation [20, 30, 31], but differentiation requires Foxn-1 [32]. The KNA/EFA [2, 9, 11] consists of mesenchyme; therefore the term EFA seems to be more appropriate than the KNA that we used [2].

4. Keratin-positive network (KPN)

The human thymic cortex shows a fine, dense keratin network that sharply differs from that of the medulla. The medulla has a loose epithelial lattice, with small, irregular-shaped EFA. A ring-shaped, anti-cytokeratin-negative "gap" of the EFA is found between the cortex and medulla (**Figures 9** and **10**) that seems to be a unique feature for the human thymus. The chicken's thymic medullary epithelial cells form a 3D network (**Figure 11**). In some places the ring-shaped "cortico-medullary gap" has small "outpocketing" toward the medulla that shows the connection of medullary EFA with the cortico-medullary gap (CMG). The medullary and cortical epithelial cells are connected, through the CMG, with epithelial bridges of medullary-type epithelial cells. In several places the CMG is not covered by the

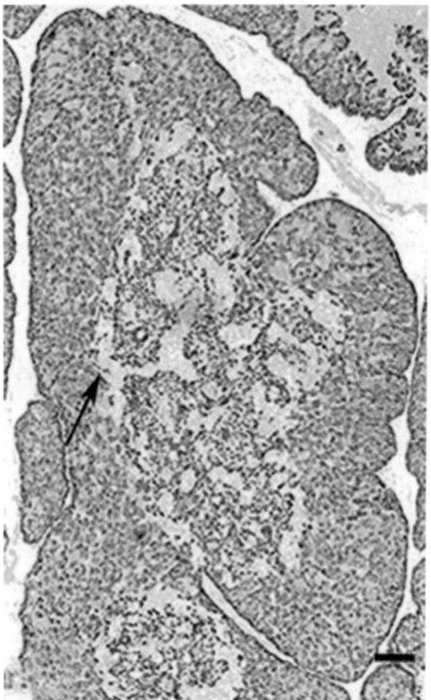

Figure 9.
Thymus 1. Age 5 months. Cortical EFA is significant compared with that of the medulla. Medullary EFA is connected with the CMG (arrow).

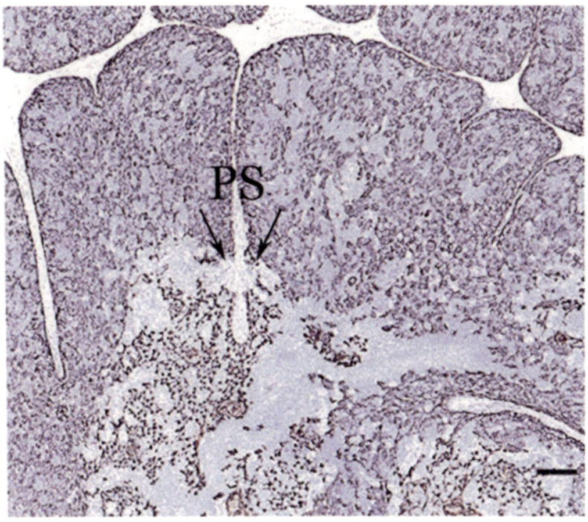

Figure 10.
Thymus 1. Age 5 months. The PS continues with the medullary EFA (arrow).

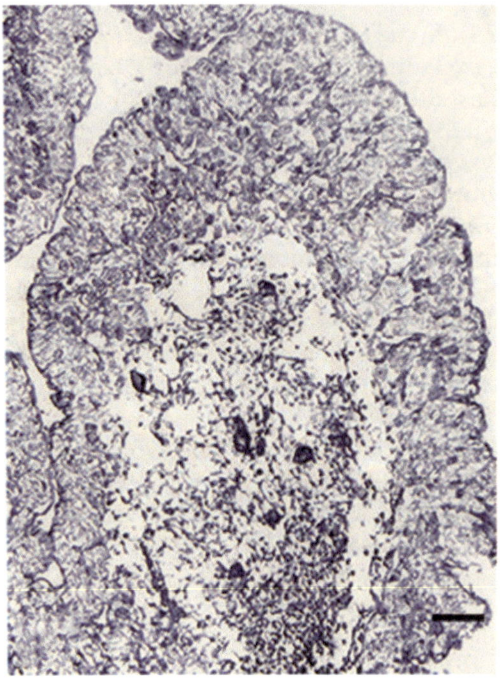

Figure 11.
Thymus 5. Age 16 months: at several places, the medullary epithelial cells, through the CMG, connect the cortex and medulla. Keratin accumulations in the medullary epithelial lattice represent Hassall's bodies.

cortex; therefore the CMG is in contact with the end of the PS. The PS reaches the CM border, widens, and become part of the medulla. Therefore, the human thymic medulla also consists of two sharply separated compartments: a keratin-positive network or lattice and an epithelium-free area. Inside the keratin-positive medullary area, few Hassall's bodies could be seen as aggregated keratin expression (**Figures 9** and **10**).

In the early embryonic life of chicken, the thymic anlage appears as a primary epithelial cord, which starts to develop from the third branchial pouch of the foregut endoderm. The epithelial cord ramifies, and this ramification area develops to medullary region of the thymus [2]. Between the offshooted secondary cords,

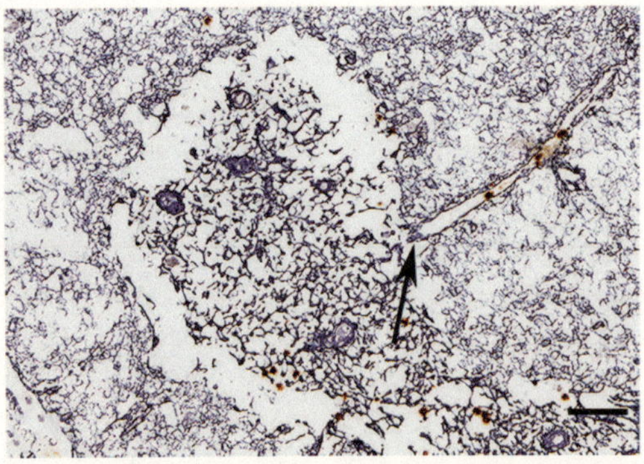

Figure 12.
Thymus 2. Age 18 months: the PS ends at the CMG (arrow). In the medulla, Hassall's bodies appear as solid, keratin-positive knots. Small keratin negative areas are also present in the cortex. The cortical surface of the gap is sharp.

the mesenchyme forms the PS and capsule (**Figure 2**). The cells at the end of the secondary cords rapidly proliferate, and by day 13, the thymic tissue is histologically recognizable (**Figure 3**). In the KPN of the medulla, several epithelial cells make large surface contact, excluding lymphocytes, from Hassall's corpuscle. It is surprising that few cells of Hassall's bodies show surfactant protein B (SPB) immunoreactivity (**Figure 12**). In the medulla, scattered SPB-positive cells also occur, which like type II pneumocytes might be developed from the foregut epithelium, that is, respiratory diverticulum.

During the last century, the origin of the thymic epithelial anlage created a hot debate: namely, the epithelial rudiment develops either from the epithelium of the endodermal pouch and ectodermal cleft or solely from the endodermal pouch. At the beginning of this century, the debate seemed to be settled: in chicken-quail chimeric experiments [26] and in mouse, transplantation of the third branchial pouch epithelium under the kidney capsule [33] proved that the pouch epithelium developed to functional thymus. Furthermore, mouse chimeras with different haplotypes of class II MHC proved that only one haplotype contributed to thymic epithelial anlage [34]. However, in human thymus the presence of a sharp CMG, among the cortex and medulla, raises again the possibility of double-germ layer origin of thymic epithelial rudiment. Bargman [35], Norris [36], and von Gaudecker [9] studied the development of human thymus and came to the conclusion that the corresponding ectodermal cleft epithelium attaches and unites with the descending third pouch epithelium (**Figure 13**). Cordier and Hamount [37] compared the thymus development of NMRI and nude mice and studied that either the lack of ectodermal cleft epithelium, which surrounded the endodermal rudiment, or the absence of a secreted substance from cleft epithelium [20] resulted in the dysgenesis of nude mouse thymus. In human thymus the major EFA is represented by the "gap" (**Figures 9** and **10**).

The debate is going on, but the subject changed over the thymic epithelial stem cell, which may be also connected to the endo- and ectodermal origin. Namely, one epithelial stem cell develops to cortical and medullary progenitors (single-germ layer origin), or there are, *sui generis*, cortical and medullary epithelial stem cells (ectodermal cleft and endodermal pouch will give raise to cortical and medullary progenitors, respectively). Between cortical and medullary microenvironment, there are many differences that also may be related to the ectodermal and endodermal origin of thymic epithelial rudiment.

The double-germ layer origin of human thymic epithelial cells is supported only by reliable histological studies and functional differences: (1) cortical epithelial

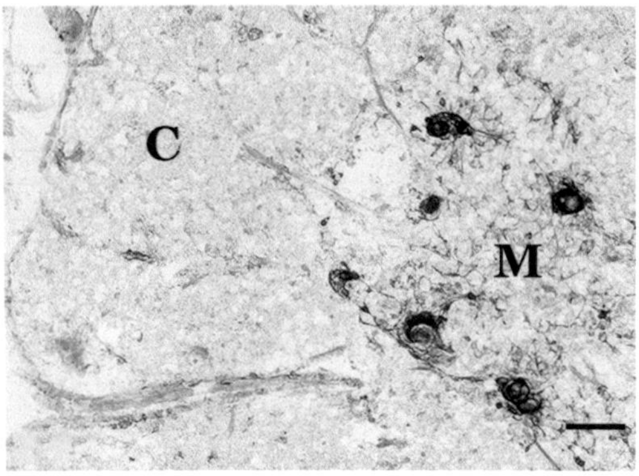

Figure 13.
Thymus 2. Age 18 months: anti-surfactant protein B (SPB) immunostaining recognizes Hassall's bodies and scattered positive cells in the medulla (M). The cortex (C) is free of SPB.

cells contribute to T-cell maturation, and the medullary ones participate in T-cell selection. (2) CMG is present in man, but not in birds and mammals studied up to now. (3) Hassall's bodies and SPB-producing cells are found only in the medulla. (4) Thymus-blood barrier exists only in the cortex [16]. (5) In the rat and mouse thymus, the cortical epithelial cells are keratin $K5^{-}$ $K8^{+}$ $CD205^{-}$, and the medullary epithelial cells are $K5^{+}$ $K8^{null}$ $CD205^{-}$ (in chicken the cortical thymic epithelial cells are $CD205^{+}$ and the medullary thymic epithelial cells are $CD205^{-}$). (6) As mentioned above thymic dysgenesis in nude mice is related with the absence of the cleft epithelium and/or cleft-derived biological active substance, which induces branchial pouch epithelial cell proliferation [31]. In mouse and chicken, the experimental data proved that the thymic epithelial anlage develops solely from the third branchial pouch [31, 33, 38–40]. The differences in the origin of epithelial anlage between man and mouse may be traced back to evolution. In marsupials there is cervical thymus, which is purely of ectodermal origin, while the cervicothoracic thymuses have mixed ecto-endodermal [37]. Evolutionary differences in organ development between man and mouse also occur: in man the allantois has rest of urachus beyond umbilicus, while in mouse the urachus is a small rudiment, and the allantois consists of pure mesenchyme [28, 41]. The relationship between thymic epithelial cells and skin keratinocytes has been supported by serological and immunofluorescence studies in normal [29, 42] and pathological conditions [3]. These investigations provide solid evidence for cross-reactive antigens among some thymic epithelial cells, cells of Hassall's corpuscles, and some subpopulation of skin keratinocytes [4].

Gupta et al. [43] studied the cytokeratin (CK5 and CK8) expression in human embryos. Before 16 weeks of gestation, the two cytokeratins are homogenously expressed in both the cortex and medulla, but after 16 weeks of gestation, the cortex and medulla show $CK8^{+}$ and $CK5^{+}$ staining, respectively. Double-positive ($CK5^{+}$ and $CK8^{+}$) epithelial progenitor cells were present only in the cortex at all gestational stages. This finding indirectly suggests that the cortex is the source of the epithelial progenitor cells. Norris [36] was able to show that the branchial cleft epithelium (cervical sinus) rapidly proliferates and surrounds the endodermal thymic rudiment. Thus, the presence of double-positive progenitor cells in the cortex and the rapid proliferation of cleft epithelium support the contribution of ectodermal component to human thymic epithelial anlage.

Hassall's bodies built up from epithelial cells. The centrally locating cells of Hassall's bodies gradually keratinized, like the epidermal cells of the skin. Neutrophil granulocytes and macrophages enter the corpuscle and digest the keratinized cells [44]. Norris [36] studied the human fetal thymuses and described migration of ectodermal cells into the medulla. This finding may be confirmed by monoclonal antibodies (mAb(s)) (RCK 105 and RGE5) which recognize cortical epithelial cells and some medullary ones [7]. These experiments may show that cortical epithelial cells enter the medulla. Furthermore, MTS29 mAb stains isolated in medullary epithelial cells. The antigen was also present in the epidermal epithelium [4]. The marginal cells of the corpuscle are alive and perhaps temporarily capable of producing SBP (**Figure 12**) and/or other biological active substances. If we adopt the double-germ layer origin of thymic epithelial cells, then both type II pneumocytes (SPB-producing cells) and the cortical stellate cells and cells of Hassall's body are in "foreign environment" of the medulla. The surface of the cell provides important information for the neighboring cell to form tissue and organs. According to the law of thermodynamic stability, if *in vitro* two types of cells are mixed and the bond among different cells is weaker than among homotypic cells, then the cells are sorting out and the homotypic cells aggregate [45]. Possibly, this is the situation *in vivo*, in case of Hassall's body formation. Several cortical cells enter the medulla and sort out, aggregating in the form of Hassall's body. The SPB-producing type II pneumocytes have got a similar situation as cortical epithelial cells; therefore the SPB-producing cells also sorting out "join" to the Hassall's bodies, resulting in SPB-positive Hassall's corpuscles [46].

5. Foxn-1 expression

Thymic epithelial cell-specific transcription factor, Foxn-1, shows scattered positive cells in both the cortex and medulla and line up along the thymic capsule and PS (**Figures 8** and **14**). The density of Foxn-1-positive cells seems to be higher in the medulla than in the cortex. Double staining with anti-cytokeratin and anti-Foxn-1 antibodies shows that Foxn-1 is expressed in both medullary compartments; namely, Foxn-1 positive cells are present in the EFA (**Figure 15**).

Acute thymic atrophy can be induced by Foxn-1 disruption [29]. Foxn-1 is necessary for the differentiation of both cortical and medullary epithelial cells [27, 47–49]. By age the number of Foxn-1-expressing epithelial cells seems to decrease [49], and this change may be paralleled with the diminished occurrence of the EFA. In elderly people, the risk of autoimmune disease is increased that may be in connection with the accumulation of Foxn-1-negative epithelial cells [49, 50] or the increased number of Foxn-1-expressing mesenchymal cells and decreased volume of EFA. However, in addition to the increasing number of Foxn-1-negative

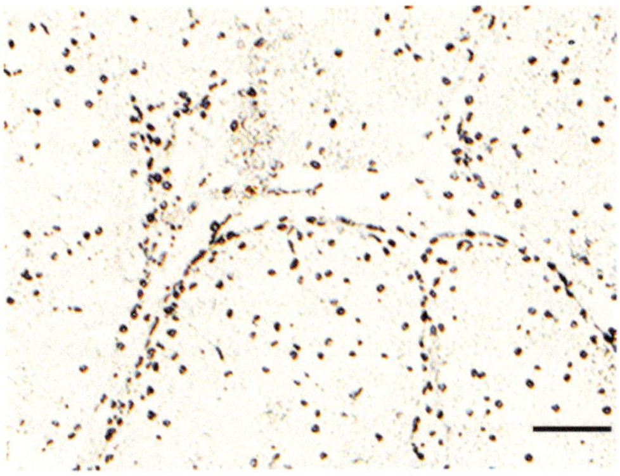

Figure 14.
Thymus 5. Age 16 months: Foxn-1-positive cells outline the thymic lobuli.

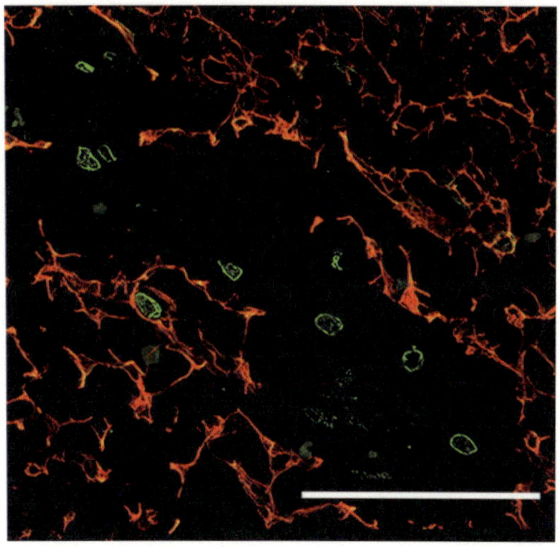

Figure 15.
Double staining: cytokeratin (red) and Foxn-1 (green). Foxn-1-positive cells are present in both the KPN and EFA of the thymic medulla.

epithelial cells, Foxn-1 is expressed in the KNA, that is, in non-epithelial cells with unknown consequences (**Figure 15**).

6. Conclusions

In the epithelium-free areas, several vessel-associated cells like pericyte and smooth-even-striated muscle cells develop from neural crest cells. It is reasonable to assume that the reticular tissue of epithelium-free area also develops from neural crest cells. In addition to this hypothesis, it is remained also unsolved if the mesenchymal cells or abnormal (keratin-free) epithelial cells express Foxn-1 transcription factor. In mouse and chicken, where the thymus develops solely from the endodermal pouch epithelium, the cortical cells enter the medulla, sort out, and

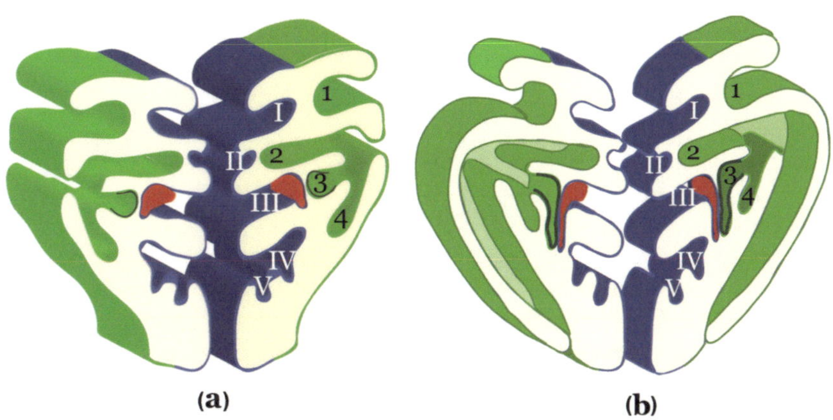

Figure 16.
Scheme: (a) from the ectodermal cervical sinus, the cervical vesicle (dark green) separates and attaches to the corresponding third branchial pouch (red), which descends into the upper mediastinum (b). (I–V, pharyngeal pouches; 1–4, pharyngeal groves). Ventral region of the third pharyngeal pouch (red) gives the endodermal part of the thymus. Part of the cervical vesicle (ectoderm, green) contributes to the thymic anlage.

form Hassall's bodies. In human thymus Hassall's corpuscles are large (compound structures), while in mouse and chicken, Hassall's bodies are small. The differences in Hassall's bodies may be related with the double- and/or single-germ layer origin of the thymic epithelial anlage (**Figure 16**).

Conflict of interest

The authors declare no conflict of interest and confirm that all these figures are original.

Abbreviations

CyA	cyclosporin A
CK	cytokeratin
CM	cortico-medullary
CMG	cortico-medullary gap
EFA	epithelium-free area
Foxn-1	Forkhead box N1
IDC	interdigitating cell
KNA	keratin negative area
KPN	keratin positive network
MHC	major histocompatibility complex
mAb	monoclonal antibody
PS	primary septum
PVS	perivascular space
SPB	surfactant protein B

Author details

Ildiko Bodi[1*], Krisztina H.-Minko[1], Zsolt Prodan[2] and Imre Olah[1]

1 Semmelweis University, Budapest, Hungary

2 Gottsegen Gyorgy Hungarian Cardiac Institute, Hungary

*Address all correspondence to: bodi.ildiko@med.semmelweis-univ.hu

References

[1] Minkó K, Oláh I. Expression of intermediate filaments and N-cadherin adhesion molecule in the thymus of domesticated birds. Acta Biologica Hungarica. 1996;**47**:323-340

[2] Bódi I, Minkó K, Molnár D, Nagy N, Oláh I. A novel aspect of the structure of the avian thymic medulla. Cell and Tissue Research. 2015;**359**:489-501. DOI: 10.1007/s00441-014-2027-1

[3] Rozing J, Coolen C, Tielen FJ, Weegenaar J, Schuurman HJ, Greiner DL, et al. Defects in the thymic epithelial stroma of diabetes prone BB rats. Thymus. 1989;**14**:125-135

[4] Godfrey DI, Izon DJ, Tucek TC, Wilson TJ, Boyd RL. The phenotypic heterogeneity of mouse thymic stromal cells. Immunology. 1990;**70**(1):66-74

[5] Schuurman HJ, van Loveren H, Rozing J, van Dijk A, Loeber JG, Vos JG. Cyclosporin and the rat thymus. An immunohistochemical study. Thymus. 1990;**16**:235-254

[6] García-Ceca J, Montero-Herradón S, Alfaro D, Zapata AG. Increased epithelial-free areas in thymuses with altered EphB-mediated thymocyte-thymic epithelial cell interactions. Histochemistry and Cell Biology. 2017;**148**:381-394. DOI: 10.1007/s00418-017-1583-3

[7] Bruijntjes JP, Kuper CF, Robinson JE, Schuurman HJ. Epithelium-free area in the thymic cortex of rats. Developmental Immunology. 1993;**3**:113-122

[8] Bódi I, Minkó K, Prodán Z, Nagy N, Oláh I. Structure of the thymus at the beginning of the 21th century. Orvosi Hetilap. 2019;**160**:163-171

[9] von Gaudecker B. The development of the human thymus microenvironment. Current Topics in Pathology. 1986;**75**:1-41

[10] Kendall MD. The morphology of perivascular spaces in the thymus. Thymus. 1989;**13**:157-164

[11] Savino W, Carnaud C, Luan JJ, Bach JF, Dardenne M. Characterization of the extracellular matrix-containing giant perivascular spaces in the NOD mouse thymus. Diabetes. 1993;**42**:134-140

[12] Mori K, Itoi M, Tsukamoto N, Kubo H, Amagai T. The perivascular space as a path of hematopoietic progenitor cells and mature T cells between the blood circulation and the thymic parenchyma. International Immunology. 2007;**19**:745-753

[13] Bryson JL, Griffith AV, Hughes B, Saito F, Takahama Y, Richie ER, et al. Cell-autonomous defects in thymic epithelial cells disrupt endothelial-perivascular cell interactions in the mouse thymus. PLoS One. 2013;**4**(8):e65196. DOI: 10.1371/journal.pone.0065196

[14] Gordon J, Bennett AR, Blackburn CC, Manley NR. Gcm2 and Foxn1 mark early parathyroid- and thymus-specific domains in the developing third pharyngeal pouch. Mechanisms of Development. 2001;**103**:141-143

[15] Gallo V, Cirillo E, Giardino G, Pignata C. FOXN1 deficiency: From the discovery to novel therapeutic approaches. Journal of Clinical Immunology. 2017;**37**:751-758. DOI: 10.1007/s10875-017-0445-z

[16] Raviola E, Karnovsky MJ. Evidence for a blood-thymus barrier using electron-opaque tracers. The Journal of Experimental Medicine. 1972;**136**:466-498

[17] W S, Boitard C, Bach JF, Dardenne M. Studies on the thymus in

nonobese diabetic mouse. I. Changes in the microenvironmental compartments. Laboratory Investigation. 1991;**64**:405-417

[18] Sawanobori Y, Ueta H, Dijkstra CD, Park CG, Satou M, Kitazawa Y, et al. Three distinct subsets of thymic epithelial cells in rats and mice defined by novel antibodies. PLoS One. 2014;**9**(10):e109995. DOI: 10.1371/journal.pone.0109995

[19] Bockman DE, Kirby ML. Dependence of thymus development on derivatives of the neural crest. Science. 1984;**223**(4635):498-500

[20] Anderson G, Jenkinson WE, Jones T, Parnell SM, Kinsella FA, White AJ, et al. Establishment and functioning of intrathymic microenvironments. Immunological Reviews. 2006;**209**:10-27. DOI: 10.1111/j.0105-2896.2006.00347.x

[21] Foster K, Sheridan J, Veiga-Fernandes H, Roderick K, Pachnis V, Adams R, et al. Contribution of neural crest-derived cells in the embryonic and adult thymus. Journal of Immunology. 2008;**180**:3183-3189

[22] Müller SM, Stolt CC, Terszowski G, Blum C, Amagai T, Kessaris N, et al. Neural crest origin of perivascular mesenchyme in the adult thymus. Journal of Immunology. 2008;**180**:5344-5351

[23] Törő I, Oláh I. Penetration of thymocytes into the blood circulation. Journal of Ultrastructure Research. 1967;**17**:439-451

[24] Lyampert IM, Beletskaya LV, Borodiyuk NA, Gnezditskaya EV, Rassokhina II, Danilova TA. A cross-reactive antigen of thymus and skin epithelial cells common with the polysaccharide of group A streptococci. Immunology. 1976;**31**:47-55

[25] Zeisberg M, Neilson EG. Biomarkers for epithelial-mesenchymal transitions. The Journal of Clinical Investigation. 2009;**119**:1429-1437. DOI: 10.1172/JCI36183

[26] Le Lièvre CS, Le Douarin NM. Mesenchymal derivatives of the neural crest: Analysis of chimaeric quail and chick embryos. Journal of Embryology and Experimental Morphology. 1975;**34**:125-154

[27] Romano R, Palamaro L, Fusco A, Iannace L, Maio S, Vigliano I, et al. From murine to human nude/SCID: The thymus, T-cell development and the missing link. Clinical & Developmental Immunology. 2012;**2012**:467101. DOI: 10.1155/2012/467101

[28] Bredenkamp N, Ulyanchenko S, O'Neill KE, Manley NR, Vaidya HJ, Blackburn CC. An organized and functional thymus generated from FOXN1-reprogrammed fibroblasts. Nature Cell Biology. 2014;**16**(9):902-908. DOI: 10.1038/ncb3023

[29] Shinohara T, Honjo T. Studies in vitro on the mechanism of the epithelial/mesenchymal interaction in the early fetal thymus. European Journal of Immunology. 1997;**27**:522-529. DOI: 10.1002/eji.1830270225

[30] Jenkinson WE, Jenkinson EJ, Anderson G. Differential requirement for mesenchyme in the proliferation and maturation of thymic epithelial progenitors. The Journal of Experimental Medicine. 2003;**198**:325-332. DOI: 10.1084/jem.20022135

[31] Jenkinson WE, Rossi SW, Parnell SM, Jenkinson EJ, Anderson G. PDGFRalpha-expressing mesenchyme regulates thymus growth and the availability of intrathymic niches. Blood. 2007;**109**:954-960. DOI: 10.1182/blood-2006-05-023143

[32] Su DM, Navarre S, Oh WJ, Condie BG, Manley NR. A domain of Foxn1 required for crosstalk-dependent thymic epithelial cell differentiation. Nature Immunology. 2003;**4**:1128-1135. DOI: 10.1038/ni983

[33] Gordon J, Wilson VA, Blair NF, Sheridan J, Farley A, Wilson L, et al. Functional evidence for a single endodermal origin for the thymic epithelium. Nature Immunology. 2004;**5**:546-553. DOI: 10.1038/ni1064

[34] Rodewald HR. Thymus organogenesis. Annual Review of Immunology. 2008;**26**:355-388. DOI: 10.1146/annurev.immunol.26.021607.090408

[35] Bargmann W. Der Thymus. In: Von Möllendorf W, editor. Blutgefäße- und Lymphgefäßapparat. Innersekretorische Drüsen, Handbuch der microskopischen Anatomie des Menschen. Vol. 6/4. Berlin, 172: Springer; 1943. p. 1

[36] Norris EH. The morphogenesis and histogenesis of the thymus gland in man: In which the origin of the Hassall's corpuscles of the human thymus is discovered. Contributions to Embryology. 1938;**27**:191-221

[37] Cordier AC, Hamount SA. Development of thymus, parathyroids and ultimo-branchial bodies in NMRI and nude mice. The American Journal of Anatomy. 1980;**157**:227-263. DOI: 10.1002/aja.1001570303

[38] Anderson G, Ritter MA. One for all and all for one: Thymic epithelial stem cells and regeneration. Trends in Immunology. 2002;**23**(8):391-395

[39] Blackburn CC, Manley NR. Developing a new paradigm for thymus organogenesis. Nature Reviews. Immunology. 2004;**4**(4):278-289

[40] Odaka C. Localization of mesenchymal cells in adult mouse thymus: Their abnormal distribution in mice with disorganization of thymic medullary epithelium. The Journal of Histochemistry and Cytochemistry. 2009;**57**:373-382. DOI: 10.1369/jhc.2008.952895

[41] Inman KE, Downs KM. The murine allantois: Emerging paradigms in development of the mammalian umbilical cord and its relation to the fetus. Genesis. 2007;**45**:237-258. DOI: 10.1002/dvg.20281

[42] Didierjean L, Saurat JH. Epidermis and thymus. Similar antigenic properties in Hassall's corpuscle and subsets of keratinocytes. Clinical and Experimental Dermatology. 1980;**5**:395-404

[43] Gupta R, Gupta T, Kaur H, Sehgal S, Aggarwal A, Kapoor K, et al. Cytokeratin (CK5, CK8, CK14) expression and presence of progenitor stem cells in human fetal thymuses. Clinical Anatomy. 2016;**29**(6):711-717. DOI: 10.1002/ca.22736

[44] Oláh I, Röchlich P, Törő I. Ultrastructure of Lymphoid Organs: An Electron-Microscopic Atlas. Budapest, Philadelphia, Toronto, Masson, Paris: Akadémiai Kiadó, J. B. Lippincott Co.; 1975

[45] Steinberg MS. Does differential adhesion govern self-assembly processes in histogenesis? Equilibrium configurations and the emergence of a hierarchy among populations of embryonic cells. The Journal of Experimental Zoology. 1970;**173**:395-433. DOI: 10.1002/jez.1401730406

[46] Steinberg MS. Differential adhesion in morphogenesis: A modern view. Current Opinion in Genetics & Development. 2007;**17**:281-286

[47] Cheng L, Guo J, Sun L, Fu J, Barnes PF, Metzger D, et al. Postnatal

tissue-specific disruption of transcription factor FoxN1 triggers acute thymic atrophy. The Journal of Biological Chemistry. 2010;**285**: 5836-5847. DOI: 10.1074/jbc. M109.072124

[48] Itoi M, Tsukamoto N, Amagai T. Expression of Dll4 and CCL25 in Foxn1-negative epithelial cells in the post-natal thymus. International Immunology. 2007;**19**:127-132

[49] Palamaro L, Romano R, Fusco A, Giardino G, Gallo V, Pignata C. FOXN1 in organ development and human diseases. International Reviews of Immunology. 2014;**33**:83-93. DOI: 10.3109/08830185.2013.870171

[50] Rode I, Martins VC, Küblbeck G, Maltry N, Tessmer C, Rodewald HR. Foxn1 protein expression in the developing, aging, and regenerating thymus. Journal of Immunology. 2015;**195**:5678-5687. DOI: 10.4049/ jimmunol.1502010

Chapter 3

Microarchitecture of the Thymus Gland; Its Age and Disease-Associated Morphological Alterations, and Possible Means to Prolong Its Physiological Activity

Arbab Sikandar, Shahzaib and Naeem Ullah

Abstract

Thymus is a ductless, highly organized, bilobed encapsulated gland of the lymphoid organs that contributes in thymopoiesis. Thymus plays an important function in the assortment, progress and profusion of T cells. The mature subsets of thymus dependent lymphocytes linked with the thymic epithelial and other cells developed the microstructure that protect the body from the harmful foreign micro-organism. Most of the thymic lobular areas experienced the parenchymal cells hypoplasia, undergone infiltration of stromal FCT and experienced thymic atrophy with age progression. As the host gets adult, the regression of the thymus and the thymopoiesis occurs, which ultimately boost the vulnerable situations of the host and open a gateway to autoimmune diseases. Since past decades, scientists are intensely investigated to develop some tactics for the improvements of the thymus performance including T-cell regeneration and maturation with age progression. This unique organ is continuously altered morphologically with age and disease; however, this microarchitectural alteration and its possible modulations is not yet clear. Therefore, the main purpose of this chapter is to highlight the microstructural compartments and physiological modification of the thymus with age. Also, the chapter is suggesting the possible alternative ways to improve its durable physio-morphology in vertebrates.

Keywords: thymus lobules, histophysiology, lymphocytes, atrophy

1. Introduction

Thymus gland is a primary lymphoid organ, situated in thoracic cavity, ascends from the endodermal layer of the third pharyngeal pouch of the embryo. Based on same origin, thymus can be linked with that of the parathyroid, but during embryogenesis it is separated from that endocrine gland [1]. Thymus faced the process of evolutionary atrophy with age in almost all the animals which leads to the architectural alterations [2]. Its anatomy is variable among species. In new-born fowl, its color is greyish pink and has two left and right lobes. It is ventral to the trachea and the large vessels, but its lobules may prolong up toward the thyroid gland.

Thymus gland in dog is a compressed bilobed structure located in the cranial mediastinum that is laying cranial to the heart and behind the sternum. Its size is largest in young which is followed by atrophy with the age progression until only a trace remains [3]. When it is fully developed, its caudal part is melded on the cranial surface of pericardium. Divisions of the inferior thyroid, internal thoracic arteries, and superior thyroid artery supply blood to the thymus. These arteries travel along the connective tissue septa, which is extended from the covering capsule into the thymic parenchyma [2]. Histologically, however, it is an old technique, but it is still used excessively in the medical field for the understanding of the organ's microarchitecture [4]. The septa divide the parenchyma into small incomplete microscopic lobules, Where they entered the thymus gland. Veins, inferior thyroid, internal thoracic and left brachiocephalic vein takes blood away from thymus gland. Nerve supply of the thymus gland arises from the sympathetic nerves of the cervical chain and the vagus nerve. Extended divisions of the phrenic nerves stretch up to the covering capsule of the thymus but are not arrive to the gland parenchyma [3]. The function of such enervations to the thymus gland is not well comprehended. Lymphatic vessels drain into the lymph nodes viz. parasternal, tracheobronchial, and brachiocephalic. Histologically, the thymus gland appears as a lobulated lymphoid organ, enclosed with a capsule, made up of a fibrous connective tissue (FCT). Capsule surrounding the organ have blood vessels which supply blood to the thymus gland parenchyma. The CT-composed trabeculae descended downward from the capsule, splits the thymus parenchyma into many incomplete lobules by extending into the interior of the organ [5]. These lobules consist of the following two parts: the cortex is a dark staining outer region just beneath the FCT capsule. It contains densely packed lymphocyte that is not involved in the formation of lymphatic nodules. This portion support the early thymocyte development also positively selects the major self-histocompatibility complex. This portion is very thick at the earlier age. The junctional point between the two compartments is called as corticomedullary junction. This is the specific area where the thymic precursor cells enter in the adult age and few of them differentiate into NK cells and the dendritic cells later few reached to the subcapsular sinuses. This corticomedullary area is also very clear and become blurting and even more fuzzy with the progression of age [6]. The medulla is a light staining inner/central region. Medulla contains later thymocyte differentiation to subpopulation like CD-4 and CD-8, also have fewer lymphocytes than cortex but have more epithelial reticular cells. It also has many thymic (Hassall's) corpuscles which differentiate it from other lymphoid tissues/glands [3]. The Hassall's corpuscles are variable sized ovoid structures composed of granule cells, epithelioid cells, and concentric layer of reticular cells containing keratohyalin and eosinophilic fibers. Under microscope the Hassall's corpuscles and the bubble-shaped adipose tissue appears in the area and their number increases with the age progression [7]. Medulla also shows the continuity between the lobules, because the lobules are incomplete. Thymocytes mature, downregulate, and reach the medullary regions.

Cellular components of the thymus glands comprise of emerging thymus-derived T cells (later population reached to 95%), the stromal cellular system including the microvasculature, the mesenchymal cells, the dendritic cells, and the very important thymic epithelial cells (TEC) [8]. Few macrophages are present in almost all parts of the gland but in medulla it plays important role in the apoptosis. The TEC are categorized into three key classes including cortical, medullar and subcapsular/perivascular based on localization in the thymic parenchyma. The dendritic cells are mostly found in the corticomedullary junction and in the medulla. All the aforementioned cells participated in the thymocyte function started from the receiving of the progenitor cells till its final training and maturation. During the period of advance gestation, the thymus in the fetus has unclear cortex and medullary regions, contains differentiating T cells, macrophages along with B cells and a developed CT capsule with the vasculature connection [9]. Soon after birth, the thymus develops altogether along with the cellular compartments. In the aged individuals, the involution of the thymus is initiated, which is easily seen in the histological sections in the form of thinning of the cortex as well as the haziness of the corticomedullar junctions. Thymic epithelial cell proliferation is a key player in the development of the thymus in the infant [5]. Recently, the hyperplastic proliferation of the thymic epithelial cells was observed in the transgenic lab animals. Thymic fragments of the neonates and that of the bone marrow transplant to the adult individual is also observed experimentally. It has been suggested that stem cells have the capacity to differentiate and develop the organ system of the same kind cells [10]. The progeny of the stem cells may develop the tissue directly or may differentiate into a new stem cell. It is possible to grow the stem cell in vitro, and it is needed to support these cells in the living individual. It would be a big achievement in the science, if the stem cells could possibly grow and could differentiate into the thymic cells in the thymus parenchyma like those present in the intestinal crypts, skin, and liver. In this chapter, we will focus on our current understanding about thymus architectural modulations in health and disease and its possible physiological improvement.

2. Physiology of thymus gland

Major role of the thymus gland is the training of variety of T cells that respond to the antigens. Its function is mainly regulating by the response of the cytokines and for this the equilibrium among anti-inflammatory and proinflammatory cytokines of the body is crucial. It has been observed that thymic atrophy is associated with age linked with diminished interleukin-7 expression [6]. Thymic epithelial cells are originated from a mutual bipotent ancestor and are also the main constituents in the growth of T cells in the thymic microstructure. It comprised of the two regions including the cortex TECs which is positioned in the cortical regions and the medulla TECs which is in the internal medulla. They experience a sequential progress which is organized by various signals, which later leads to support in physiological maturation and development of the thymocyte. The TECs playing a role in the selection of T- cells in the thymus parenchyma [5]. Both cortical and medullar TECs play distinctive responsibilities in the positive and negative selections of the thymocyte.

3. Differentiation, proliferation, and development of lymphocytes

The undifferentiated lymphocytes are migrated from the reservoir, that is, bone marrow to the thymus gland by means of blood stream. The thymic cortex contains the reticular cells, also known as thymic nurse cells. These cells surround the lymphocytes and enhance the differentiation, proliferation, and maturation of the cells [11]. The lymphocytes get matured and get transformed into immunocompetent cytotoxic T cells, helper T cells, and the T cell. At this stage, the receptor is being attached at surface of the lymphocytes for the recognition of antigens. This process starts just before the birth and continues till some month after the birth. Almost 1% of the mature lymphocytes are getting out of thymus toward the margin on daily basis. The differentiation and further activations of T cells to CD-4 and CD-8, and then established T cells travels from thymus to the marginal blood vessels and secondary immune organs [9, 11]. Thus, the size and mass of thymus reflect the maturation of the immune system.

4. Blood-thymus barrier

It is a physical barrier formed by endothelial cells, epithelial reticular cells, and macrophages. Its function is to prevent developing lymphocytes from the exposure of blood borne antigen [8]. This barrier provides tremendous environment for the substance exchange between vasculature and the thymus also help maturation of the immature thymocytes. Macrophages present outside the capillaries prevent the interaction of the substances that are transported in the blood vessels with the developing T cells in the cortex. Matured T cells leave the thymus gland through the blood vessels and colonize in the lymph node, spleen, and lymphatic tissue of the organism [11].

5. Maturation and selection of T cells

Maturation is the condition of developing progenitor within the thymus parenchyma, where the cells known as thymocytes, undergoes various developmental processes to perform exclusively. These cells can be recognized based on manifestation of various markers on the cell surface and the antigen presenting cells present the T cells with self and foreign antigen [11]. It usually consists of positive selection in which the lymphocytes that recognize the foreign antigens survived and reached to the maturity then enter the medulla through the cortex. Later, goes to the other sites in the body via blood [9]. Maturation is a very complicated process and only a small number of lymphocytes reach to the stage of maturity in the thymus. The negative selection in which the lymphocytes which are incapable to distinguish the self-antigens are eliminated by the macrophages. This is approximately 95% of the total cells.

6. Function of epithelial reticular cells

Epithelial reticular cells, also called as TECs, are present both in the cortex and medulla; however, it can be easily recognizable in the thymic medulla through histology. These cells contained the thymic granules which is assumed to be the called as the thymic hormone [12]. This structure has the following functions;

- It formed the blood-thymus barrier.
- Secrete hormone which are required for proliferation, differentiation, and maturation of T cells. Also, for the expression of their surface markers. The hormones including thymulin, thymopoietin, thymosin, thymic numeral factor, interleukin, and interferon are secreted.
- It forms thymic (Hassall's) corpuscles, distinctive whorls, in the medulla of the thymus gland. The thymus gland is identified by this thymic corpuscle.

The pluripotent progenitor cells migrated from the bone marrow to the thymus parenchyma, where the maturation of the unexperienced T cells occurs in the complex microarchitecture. However, this structure changes with the age.

7. Age associated changes occurs in the thymus

Aging is an irreversible, on-going, and inevitable progression that is correlated through manifold organ dysfunction. The key organ of immune system and primary organ of T cell production is the thymus gland which is endodermal in nature. Involution of the thymus with progressing age is into the consequences of a decreased T cell production primarily and leads toward a long list of the following diseases and even a mortality of the individual [6]. The corticomedullary junction is disrupted and the number of medullary epithelial cells are also decrease. This age-related cellular apoptosis and atrophy is still un-answered. There are several reasons to be considered for this process, but the main cause known is reactive oxygen species (ROS). The entity that are assumed to be responsible for expressing the age-related changes in the thymus is due to the discrepancy amongst the free oxygen-derived radicles and that of the antioxidants. Mitochondria is the main site were such reactive species are produced. Inside mitochondria, the oxidative stress produce ROS which results into mitochondrial damage within the cells and leads to liberate more ROS. In fact, aging is a physiological multifactorial process accompanied by decline of organ function. Histologically, the thymus gland of mammals divided into three consecutive morphological stages; the epithelial, the lymphopoietic, and the differentiated cellular microenvironment [7]. The progenitor cells are synthesizing in the thymus which later differentiated into mature T cells. Thymus also comprises the main stromal niche termed as thymic epithelial space. It supports T cell development and maturation [6]. The thymus is greater in size and is very dynamic in the neonates and pre-adolescents. With the progression in age, the involution starts and ultimately disappears and are then replaced by rudiments and fat. The process of involution started just after 1 year of birth [2]. If in case the thymus is absent in individual congenitally, then there would be a probable chance of deficiency of T cells. The main components of the thymus which undergoes involution during the aging include the T cells of hematopoietic origin and the TECs of non-hematopoietic origin. During the process of involution, disruption of the thymic epithelial/endothelial ratio happened and results into gradual loss of pro-T cells. Primarily just after the start of involution, the thymic epithelium mass is decreased in the parenchyma. This decrease in epithelium leads toward the disorganization of corticomedullary junction and results into loss of demarcation between the thymic cortex and medulla. This process where a continuous loss of cells and their functions is called aging [6]. Histology of thymus gland varies with the individual's age. It is observed that this gland is extremely delicate to stand against the biological abnormalities, for example, autoimmune diseases, infection, and age progression. It attains its maximum development shortly after birth. After attaining the age of puberty, the thymus gland regress and degenerate. Due to this effect the lymphocyte production decreases and the reticuloepithelial cells (thymic corpuscles) increases. Cellular portion, especially of T cell of thymus gland, decreases and are being replaced by connective tissue and adipose cells. Parenchyma of the thymus gland at and after puberty is filled with adipose tissue. Immunity, however, in this stage it is not compromised because progeny of the T lymphocytes has already been established. Thymus gland is well developed only in late fetal life and persists for a few months after birth [6]. Subsequent to this period, it undergoes rapid atrophy, fatty infiltration, and the amyloid degeneration [13]. Increase in the amount of adipose tissue and fat-bearing cells in the thymus parenchyma indicates that the body is now vulnerable to the infection and autoimmune diseases. So, in adult, only a thin remnant appeared in the anterior mediastinum or has entirely disappeared. Thymus gland size is also affected by the sex-steroid hormone and hypothalamic-pituitary-adrenal axes hormones [14]. It has been found that during the thymus involution, the CT which is present in the capsule, septa, perivascular tissue, and in the stroma of the cortex and medulla is getting enriched with the fibronectin contents. Later, most of the thymic parenchymal areas are being replaced by the stromal cells.

8. Effect of removal of the thymus gland and its clinical significance

Thymus gland is an important component of immune system. This system defends the host from several infections [11]. It's inappropriate performance may produce embarrassment or even fatality. If the thymus gland is removed from the new borne individual, then there will be no possibility of the T cell production [6]. Other, lymphoid organs will also lack or decrease the number of T cell to fight against the pathogens. Consequently, death of the individual may occur, predominantly due to complications with infection and lack of immunity.

9. Effect of malfunctioning thymus gland on the body

Thymus experiences atrophy with time which is triggered by numerous factors viz. growth and aging, infections and endocrine instabilities which give rise to a nonstandard liberation of T cells and consequently weakened the immunity [6]. The main organic task of this gland is to spawn a distinct T cells range to establish a crucial portion in host immunity counter to external pathogens, whereas the thymus correspondingly theaters a serious part in self-tolerance through negative assortment and the T reg cells formerly known as suppresser T cells production. Some of the thymic-derived malfunctionings are categorized bellow.

9.1 Hypersensitivity/immunodeficiency or autoimmune disease

When the immune system of body trigger against its own body cells and show the excessive action then the allergic condition developed [15]. Allergens are the substances which initiate the allergic response. IgE antibodies are more common in this condition. Histamine is also present in allergic condition which are released from the Mast cells. Anaphylaxis is a condition developed when these allergens cause an acute to severe reaction and that sometimes proves fatal condition. In this case, the immune system becomes hyperactive and cause the death of own host cells instead of killing foreign pathogens. Thymus parenchymal cells have the ability to recognition the body own cells and prevent them from killing central tolerance process that is immunologic tolerance to self-antigens. During such diseases, the demarcation between the cortex and the medulla deteriorated and the medullar epithelial cells are also dispersed [16]. A rare autoimmune polyendocrinopathy-candidiasis-ectodermal dystrophy is an inherited syndrome and is because of alterations in the specific gene [14]. Such gene permits the illustration of tissue related particular proteins present in the thymic medulla. This disease also affects multiple endocrine tissues. As T cell production take place in the thymus gland and if there is any defect in thymocyte development, it leads to profound decrease in the production of T cell, which may result into immunodeficiency disease. Abnormality to the thymic epithelial cells leads to the T cells dysfunctions, which may result in chronic inflammatory disease in the host [11, 12]. The tolerance is failed due to available antigens in the tissue is because of the autoimmune illnesses. If there is a defect in the production of both T cell and B cell, it results into severe combined immunodeficiency (SCID). When the combine deficiency of T lymphocytes and B lymphocytes occurs together, then the condition developed is known as SCID. This is a rare congenital disease, which is initiated by the non-functional hematopoietic progenitor cells that act as precursor of the B lymphocytes and T lymphocytes. When this condition develops, there is decrease in the lymphocytes production which results into the thymus atrophy [16]. There are also some other factors which are responsible for the causation of this disease such as IL-7 deficiency, recombination activating gene deficiency and common gamma chain deficiency. Another autoimmune disease in which the antibodies blocks the acetylcholine receptors at neuromuscular junction. This autoimmune disease is known as myasthenia gravis. This illness is categorized as softness and fatigability of the muscle and is triggered by autoantibodies depending T cell counter to the neuromuscular junction. Its exact cause is unknown; however, it is assumed that changes in the thymus and the thymic epithelial cells is one of the main causes of its pathogenesis [14, 15]. Sometimes, this disease is associated with thymic hyperplasia. This disease is commonly cured by the surgical amputation of the thymus which is known as thymectomy. The conditions like thymic hyperplasia or malignancy are nearly 70% more common in the patients suffering with such autoimmune disease. Type-1 diabetes is also an autoimmune-based disease, which results from the obliteration of β cells in the islets of Langerhans. The pancreas infiltrating T lymphocytes cause the destruction of the insulin producing cells in the islets of Langerhans. The body, in this case, does not produce insulin. It is seemed to be more commonly present in adults. It has been observed that lack of immune tolerance to the β cells present in the pancreas is the initial cause of such diabetes development. The Human immunodeficiency virus (HIV virus) effect the developing lymphocytes and results into killing of these cells [18]. When the lymphocytes decrease in the body, then the T cell immunodeficiency syndrome occurs, which are acquired in nature. The HIV virus usually cause the killing the CD4 T cells and it also mainly effect the mature T lymphocytes which are present at the periphery. In this case, a rapid atrophy of the thymus takes place in the infected individual.

9.2 DiGeorge syndrome

This inherited ailment is because of the obliteration of a minor piece of chromosome-22, which is one of 23 pair of human chromosomes [17]. The syndrome affects the individual through various means like cleft palate, facial defects, delay development, learning problems, and promote infections. As far as the immunity is concerned, this syndrome leads to inherited shortcomings containing thymic atrophy and aplasia. Such affected persons may have intense deficiency of T cell lineage. In this disease, the thymic parenchymal cells are lost and the area is then replaced by the stromal CT.

9.3 Tumors

Thymomas is a scarce neoplasia (benign in nature) arise from the thymic epithelial cells. In the thymoma patients, there are chances for the occurrence of a disease known as thymoma-associated multiorgan autoimmunity (TAMA). In these patients, the donor does not act like a basis of pathogenic T cells instead, the individual particular thymus gland yields the infected T cells which is directed toward its own body cells [19]. If the thymoma indicates the malignancy of the thymus gland, then its product is the defective T cells which are unable to recognize their own body cells as self-antigens. So that is why we can hardly distinguish this disease from GVHD. These types of tumors, usually 10–15%, are presented in the patients who are already suffering from myasthenia gravis. The symptoms include strong cough which sometimes get confused with bronchitis because the laryngeal nerve is compressed by the tumor. All thymomas are cancerous, but they are varied from each other in different aspects like some develop slowly and some tumors grow with the rapid rate and infect the surrounding tissue [20]. The treatment of this condition is the surgical removal of the infected part or whole gland.

Thymic lymphomas are tumors which originate from the thymocytes of the thymus gland. These lymphomas or leukemia acts like the precursors of the origin of the thymocyte are often classified as T acute lymphoblastic leukemia/lymphoma. Before 1950, the radiation was used to cure the people who are suffering from the enlarged thymus gland particularly the children. The post-operative complication in the treated people includes an elevated incidence of thyroid cancer and leukemia. The rare malformation of thymus gland includes the cervical thymus cyst which is something confusing with the tumors. In the literature, there is no as such detail study of the thymic cyst prevalence. There is no such common lesion appeared which are present in this condition. In the childhood, there are more chances of the thymic cyst and the ectopic cervical thymus than the adults.

10. Means to modulate the functioning of the thymus gland

Thymic involution with age has negative impacts on the immune system. Proper performance of the thymus and integral immune system are required to protect against disorders. With the advancements of the modern sciences, a technique named as photobiomodulation is newly employed to slower the process of thymic involution. This delayed process improves immunity and may add in extension of the individual lifespan. Another new method which reduce the thymus atrophy and boost the thymus functioning is the sex-steroid ablation therapies [14]. Genetics has also an important role for determining the initial thymus size and rate of involution. Many hormonal medications, surgical procedures, and applications of antioxidants are testified as replacements for the reversal of aging in atrophy of the thymus. Males display a trend of lower grade thymopoiesis in comparison to females. There are several procedures that can improve the normal physiology of the thymus gland which ultimately leads to strengthen the immune system active for prolong time [20]. Continuous use of dietary supplements like rosehips, echinacea, olive leaf, and cruciferous vegetables are tested to be connected to establishment of the thymus health. These supplements are comprised of glucosinolates. This substance is famous for fighting contrary to the tumorous cells and other malformations in the tissues. Vegetables especially cruciferous vegetables like cauliflower, Bok Choy, broccoli, and cabbage are good source of nutrients that trigger antioxidants and anti-inflammatory responses. This can also assist thymus function. Proper timely intake of antioxidants and various vitamins like E and C in the diet is mostly necessary. These are needed for proper functioning of the thymus cells [21]. Zinc is also a very useful micronutrient required for the growth and growth of the vertebrate. The immune system is very sensitive to zinc deficiency and produces the multiple disturbances like atrophy of the thymus parenchyma and the increased chances for a disease to occur [22]. Many genes which regulate thymus gland activity are under the response of metalloenzymes in which zinc act as metal. So, dietary supplementation is very necessary for the proper functioning of the thymus gland otherwise, there may be a serious consequence related to the synthesis of the T lymphocytes. Exercise on daily basis is additional tool to ensure blood circulation throughout the body and the thymus gland. In this way increased blood flow will ensure that thymus waste products are removed promptly and do not cause damage to the thymus. Furthermore, through the circulation the key nutrients reach around the body more rapidly which allow quicker recovery to take place. Thymus gland stimulate the production of white blood cells that help against infection by thymosin hormone. This thymus glandular extract regulates many other immune functions. The extract called as thymomodulin, obtained from bovine species and act as immune boosting activities in immunodeficient individuals. Such extract act as a substitute and work against respiratory infections and many other infections like asthma, food allergies and hay fever. Olive leaf extract has a significant effect on thymocyte apoptosis and cell cycle progression to protect the thymus gland from toxicity. Tapping sternum is a practice which may also stimulate thymus gland. But this practice is a bit laborious. Organic acid has a positive effect on the immune system. It has been reported that sodium butyrate improves the thymus histology and ultimately improves the immune system of a body [23]. Probiotics are called as the group of beneficial bacteria. Probiotics are generally defined as the friendly living micro-organ¬isms, when taken orally in an appropriate dose, exhibit a beneficial effect on the host health. When the probiotics is taken orally, they go along side of the lumen of the gastrointestinal tract and interact with the mucosal immune system. Here, the whole bacteria or its cell wall mediate a network of signal production and activate the immune system. They produce different kinds of cytokines and chemokines and result into the activation of T lymphocytes. Another model of mechanism of action of probiotics is that they can suppress the growth of pathogenic bacteria and help in the balancing of microflora environment in the gastrointestinal tract. Probiotics protect the body against the pathogens by the induction of direct killing, nutritional competency of pathogens, and meanwhile by triggering the gut-associated immune repertoire. Thymus gland is known as the "Master gland of immunity" [2]. It regulates the immune system by producing different types of chemical known as cytokines that enhance the migration of T lymphocytes and meantime enhances the immunity [20]. The probiotic fermented milk (PFM) is a nutritional supplement which is used to improve the histology of the thymus gland mean to say it will cause a decrease in cellular apoptosis and enhance the percentage of CD4/CD8 cells. The PFM enhance the production of different kinds of cytokines in the thymus gland. This type of milk is usually used in case of protein-energy malnutrition; which result into malfunctioning of the immune system. This milk or bacterial-free supernatant helps to improve the immune system by activating thymus gland activity. Commonly used probiotics are specific strains of the lactic acid bacteria. The main genus includes in the probiotics are the *Bifidobacteria*, *Streptococci*, *Lactobacilli*, *Enterococcus*, *Pediococcus*, along with some yeast. Some probiotics like *L. paracasei* CNCM I-1518 and *L. casei* CRL 431 have a toll like receptors through which they make an attachment with the intestinal epithelial cells. Here, they mediate the immune stimulation by producing cytokines such as IL-6 and protein 1, which is chemoattractant in nature. Most of the probiotics are physically strengthening the intestinal barrier by producing the mucus layer, which is secreted from the goblet cells in the intestine. This viscous and impermeable mucus layers protect the intestinal barrier also stimulate the IgA and motivate the immunity. The probiotics also improve the health of animal by producing low molecular organic acids such as acetic acid and lactic acid. They also produce high molecular weight antimicrobial compound known as bacteriocins. These have strong inhibitory effect on the pathogenic gram-negative bacteria, i.e., *H. pylori* and the *Salmonella* species [24]. They inhibit the growth of pathogenic microbes and improve the health of animals. The lactobacilli containing probiotic has the ability to protect the children and adults from antibiotic-associated diarrhea and reduces its risk. *L. acidophilus* or *L. casei* are those probiotics can regulate the composition of microbial species present in the gut at balance level and suppress the growth of pathogenic bacteria. *L. acidophilus* or *L. casei* and lactic acid bacteria together act and result into suppressing the fecal coliform and other anaerobic bacteria. Some probiotics are also responsible for the shifting of microbes of gut to the beneficial bacteria, e.g., *Prevotella* and *Oscillibacter*. These bacteria are responsible for the production of anti-inflammatory metabolites. It can cause decrease the polarization of Th17 which favors the differentiation of anti-inflammatory Treg/Type 1 regulatory T (Tr1) cells in the gut. The *S. thermophilus* and *L. acidophilus* probiotics have ability to increase the intestinal integrity by enhancing the gene expression in tight junction signaling. These probiotics decrease the adhesion entero-invasive *E. coli* in HT29 and Caco-2 cells by the maintenance (actin and ZO-1) or enhancement (actinin and occludin) of cytoskeletal and tight junctional protein phosphorylation. Antimicrobial peptides produced by probiotics are now considered as the future of the new class of therapeutics because it produces lesser resistance and have a specific antimicrobial activity to protect the host. Different kinds of antimicrobial peptides like lysozyme, secretory phospholipase A2, defensins, defensin-like peptides (elafin and SLPI), and cathelicidins are produce from the paneth cells. These are the characteristics epithelial cells of the small intestinal which is located at the bottom of the intestinal crypts. The probiotics *B. subtilis* was found in improvement of the thymus microarchitecture in broilers [25]. Prebiotics are those high fibrous non-digestible food particles that are used as a source of energy for the beneficial bacteria like bifidobacteria and lactobacteria and symbiotic is the combination of the probiotics and the prebiotics. It modulates the host immune system and usually effect the intestinal microflora and regulate the immune system directly and indirectly. When symbiotic are administered during the embryo it enhances the proliferation of the lymphocytes by causing decrease in the cortex/medulla ratio of the thymus gland. In a research, a number of prebiotics like inulin (Pre1), Bi2tos (Pre2), and also a symbiotic composed of inulin and *Lactococcus lactis* subsp. lactis IBB SL1 (Syn1), a symbiotic composed of Bi2tos and *L. lactis* subsp. cremoris IBB SC1 (Syn2), is administrated in the early chick embryonic life in order to check its effect on the lymphoid tissue activity. B. longum and a prebiotic (Synergy 1) when administered into the body, can enhance the release of defensins from epithelial cells and they have antimicrobial activity. The outcomes of the research come in the form of enhance lymphocytes proliferation. When the Bi2tos were administered with *L. lactis* subsp. cremoris (Syn2) they caused reduction of the thymic cortex to medullary ratio [26]. This indicates the more spreading of the medulla without the effect on the cortex representing the subsequent impacts on the thymus.

11. Conclusion

The thymus is a part of primary immune organs, having excellent example of connection between the cellular organization and function. Not like other well-organized organs, the microstructure of the thymus parenchyma has the very complex meshwork, where T cells differentiate, proliferate, and die. Disorganized thymic architecture of the elderly and disease thymus added cavitation and FCT proliferation and atrophy. Moreover, defects in the thymus caused to lesser the production of T cells and the interruption of self-tolerance. This may result in worsening the development of disease. Consequently, the thymus is declared as one of the most significant organs in maintaining immunity and safeguard the host against progression of age and development of ailments. Subsequently, this gland acts a crucial part in health and disease. The size, architecture, and function of this gland decreases with progression of age. There are some possible pathways to modify the thymus microarchitecture and function, in order to progress the physiology during autoimmune diseases, infections, and aging.

Author details

Arbab Sikandar*, Shahzaib and Naeem Ullah
Sub-Campus, Jhang, University of Veterinary and Animal Sciences, Lahore, Pakistan

*Address all correspondence to: arbab.sikandar@uvas.edu.pk; drarbab786@gmail.com

References

[1] Wilson M, Coyle M. Embryology of the branchial arches. In: Clinical Embryology. Cham: Springer; 2019. pp. 169-176

[2] Geenen V, Wilson S. History of the thymus: From a vestigial organ to the programming of immunological self-tolerance. In: Thymus Transcriptome and Cell Biology. Cham: Springer; 2019. pp. 1-18

[3] Kalhor N, Cesar M. The thymus: Practical anatomy and histology. In: Mediastinal Pathology. Cham: Springer; 2019. pp. 1-12

[4] Sikandar A. Histopathology: An old yet important technique in modern science. In: Histopathology-an Update. IntechOpen; 2018

[5] Sakata M, Izumi O, Yousuke T. Cellularity of thymic epithelial cells in the postnatal mouse. The Journal of Immunology. 2018;**200**(4):1382-1388

[6] Thomas R, Dong-Ming S. Age-related thymic atrophy: Mechanisms and outcomes. In: Thymus. IntechOpen; 2019

[7] Gouse H, Suban M, Suban MG, Gunasegaran JP. Histological and histometrical study on human fetal thymus. Health Sciences. 2019;**8**(3):90-109

[8] Hirakawa M, Daisuke N, Benoît K, Sergiy A, Brigitte K, Christiane H, et al. Fundamental parameters of the developing thymic epithelium in the mouse. Scientific Reports. 2018;**8**(1):11095

[9] Zhang L, Zimo Z, Hao M, Baoliang L, Bin W, Ling Y. Modulation of helper T cytokines in thymus during early pregnancy in ewes. Animals. 2019;**9**(5):245

[10] Zhan Y, Lihua W, Guangyang L, Xiaohui Z, Jingci Y, Yuxia P, et al. The reparative effects of human adipose-derived mesenchymal stem cells in the chemotherapy-damaged thymus. Stem Cells and Development. 2019;**28**(3):186-195

[11] Shortman K, Heather J. The differentiation of T lymphocytes: I. proliferation kinetics and interrelationships of subpopulations of mouse thymus cells. Cellular Immunology. 1974;**12**(2):230-246

[12] Mandel T. Differentiation of epithelial cells in the mouse thymus. Zeitschrift für Zellforschung und Mikroskopische Anatomie. 1970;**106**(4):498-515

[13] Taub DD, Longo DL. Insights into thymic aging and regeneration. Immunological Reviews. 2005;**205**(1):72-93

[14] Leposavić GM, Pilipović IM. Intrinsic and extrinsic thymic adrenergic networks: Sex steroid-dependent plasticity. Frontiers in Endocrinology. 2018;**9**:13

[15] Benn CS, Jeppesen DL, Hasselbalch H, Olesen AB, Nielsen J, Björkstén B, et al. Thymus size and head circumference at birth and the development of allergic diseases. Clinical & Experimental Allergy. 2001;**31**(12):1862-1866

[16] Myers LA, Patel DD, Puck JM, Buckley RH. Hematopoietic stem cell transplantation for severe combined immunodeficiency in the neonatal period leads to superior thymic output and improved survival. Blood. 2002;**99**(3):872-878

[17] Markert ML, Boeck A, Hale LP, Kloster AL, McLaughlin TM, Batchvarova MN, et al. Transplantation of thymus tissue in complete DiGeorge

syndrome. New England Journal of Medicine. 1999;**341**(16):1180-1189

[18] Savino W, Dardenne M, Marche C, Trophilme D, Dupuy JM, Pekovic D, et al. Thymic epithelium in AIDS. An immunohistologic study. The American Journal of Pathology. 1986;**122**(2):302

[19] Rosai J. Histological Typing of Tumours of the Thymus. Berlin, Heidelberg: Springer-Verlag, Springer Science & Business Media; 2012

[20] Thomson AD, Thackray AC. The histology of tumours of the thymus. British Journal of Cancer. 1957;**11**(3):348

[21] Good RA. Nutrition and immunity. Journal of Clinical Immunology. 1981;**1**(1):3-11

[22] Hidayat C, Jayanegara A, Wina E. Effect of zinc addition on the immune response and production performance of broilers: A meta-analysis. Asian-Australasian Journal of Animal Sciences. 2019. Available from: https://www.ajas.info/journal/view.php?doi=10.5713/ajas.19.0146

[23] Sikandar A, Zaneb H, Younus M, Masood S, Aslam A, Khattak F, et al. Effect of sodium butyrate on performance, immune status, microarchitecture of small intestinal mucosa and lymphoid organs in broiler chickens. Asian-Australasian Journal of Animal Sciences. 2017a;**30**(5):690

[24] Sikandar A, Zaneb H, Younus M, Masood S, Aslam A, Ashraf S, et al. Protective effect of sodium butyrate on growth performance, immune responses and gut mucosal morphometry in salmonella-challenged broiler chickens. International Journal of Agriculture and Biology. 2017b;**19**(6):1387-1393

[25] Sikandar A, Zaneb H, Younus M, Masood S, Aslam A, Shah M, et al. Growth performance, immune status and organ morphometry in broilers fed Bacillus subtilis-supplemented diet. South African Journal of Animal Science. 2017;**47**(3):378-388

[26] Madej JP, Stefaniak T, Bednarczyk M. Effect of in ovo-delivered prebiotics and synbiotics on lymphoid-organs' morphology in chickens. Poultry Science. 2015;**94**(6):1209-1219

Chapter 4

Thymic Senescence

Krisztian Kvell

Abstract

Thymic senescence develops in every person, although at different pace. Thymic senescence significantly lowers the production of naive T cells, leading to increased incidence of infections, cancer and autoimmune diseases. Certain external factors can accelerate thymic senescence. These include chemicals (copper-chelators), hormones (androgens), infections (viruses, fungi, protozoa). Others may slow the aging process of the thymus including perturbations to the hormonal (sex-steroid) system, genetic alterations (PPARgamma deficiency) or chemical compounds (PPARgamma antagonists). Thymic senescence research may provide insight to underlying molecular events and potentially appoint novel therapeutic targets for senescence intervention strategies. These hold promise to postpone thymus senescence and enhance T cell production. That would result in a decreased incidence of infections, cancer and autoimmune diseases, currently affecting the elderly. The attributed drop in healthcare costs and gain in quality of life share tremendous economic and social interest.

Keywords: thymus, senescence, adipose tissue

1. The aging thymus

Transcription factor TBX-1 is a mastermind in the formation of the third pharyngeal pouch involved in thymus organogenesis during embryonic development [1]. Patients with 22q11.2DS that impairs TBX-1 often present thymus hypoplasia. Similarly, Tbx-1^{null} mice develop hypoplasia of the thymus [2, 3]. In both cases, defective thymus organogenesis leads to impaired thymocyte development [4]. However, as reported recently, the role of TBX-1 in thymus organogenesis is not straightforward. Ectopic forced expression of TBX-1 can inhibit transcription factor FoxN1, the mastermind of thymic epithelial identity thus indirectly impair thymus identity via sustained presence [5]. The thymus contains developing T cells (aka thymocytes) along with the non-lymphoid thymic stromal elements comprising the microenvironment that promotes thymocyte differentiation. Stromal elements include thymic epithelial cells (aka TECs), mesenchymal cells, endothelial cells as well as non-lymphoid hematopoietic cells (e.g., dendritic cells or macrophages). TECs constitute the main functional stromal cell type necessary to promote thymocyte differentiation [6, 7]. Soon after birth the thymus expands to increase the output of naive T cells, in order to colonize available niches in the periphery [8–10]. Cortical TECs (aka cTECs) are required for T lineage commitment, along with thymocyte expansion and differentiation, and positive selection. Medullary TECs (mTECs) are necessary for the induction of central tolerance and subsequent stages of thymocyte maturation before leaving the thymus. Of note, in order to maintain the well organized cortical and medullary compartments active (reverse) intercellular signaling is also required from developing thymocytes towards TECs

IntechOpen

(aka cross-talk) [11, 12]. At a vaguely defined time point, the thymus begins to show involution, resulting in adipose degeneration of the organ; hence the process termed adipose involution. This senescent process is accompanied by the stepwise disorganization of thymic compartments, also shifting TEC subset ratios and reducing naive T cell production. Although the detailed mechanisms triggering these processes remain to be fully elucidated, they finally deteriorate thymus structure and function, severely impairing the output of fresh naive T cells. Decline of fresh naive T cells results in the inverse increase of memory T cell representation due to aging [13–15]. The observed bias in cTEC:mTEC ratio, and the fading of the most differentiated MHC class II-expressing TEC subsets leads to the development of a less complex medullary architecture along with the blurring of the cortico-medullary junction. This is followed by the focal disappearance of epithelial cells, gradually being replaced by adipose tissue in the perivascular spaces [16–20]. There is mounting evidence that adipose cells may have an thymic origin. Thymic adipose cells also produce an array of cytokines and signaling molecules that directly affect (impair) thymopoiesis [21–25]. As a result, although the appearance of thymic adipocytes may not trigger involution, their increasing presence with senescence can indirectly facilitate or perhaps even directly deteriorate thymus function. Thymus involution likely develops as a sum of failure of thymocyte progenitors and the inappropriate function of TEC compartments. It has been reported that the number of early T lineage precursors (aka ETPs) shows a gradual decline with senescence [26]. Reconstitution experiments of senescent thymi with bone marrow precursors from young donors cannot restore thymic compartments nor rescue impaired thymopoiesis. The opposite, however, reconstitution of young recipients using senescent bone marrow cells does not impair thymopoiesis [27, 28]. The genetic inactivation of cell cycle inhibitor p27 (aka Cdkn1b) also leads to the development of an enlarged thymus and enhances fresh naive T cell output along with normal stromal organization [29–33]. Recent thymic emigrants (aka RTEs) show a decrease upon enhanced expression of LIF, SCF, IL-6, and M-CSF [34, 35].

2. Characterization of thymic adipose tissue

There are significant differences between adipose tissue subtypes. At least three subtypes are distinguished: white adipose tissue (WAT), brown adipose tissue (BAT) and the recently described beige adipose tissue. White adipose tissue stores energy, brown adipose tissue generates heat (via NST or non-shivering thermogenesis), while beige adipocytes act as intermediates. It has currently been described that thymic adipose involution yields beige adipose tissue based on its gene expression, miRNA, histology and metabolic profile [36]. In terms of gene expression and histology characteristic epithelial markers show down-regulation (FoxN1, EPCAM1, MHCII, Wnt4) (see **Figure 1**). Considering the miRNA profile beige-adipose tissue-associated miRNA species show supportive changes (miR27a, miR106b, miR155) (see **Figure 1**). While PPARgamma is the mastermind of all adipose tissue subtypes, TBX-1 has been acknowledged as a key and specific marker of beige adipose tissue development [17–20]. Beige adipocytes respond to adrenergic stimuli by thermogenesis via mitochondrial uncoupling of biochemical degradation and energy production [21]. Along with TBX-1 other beige-indicative markers have also been reported. These include mitochondrial uncoupling proteins (mostly UCP-1), EAR2 (also known as Nr2f6) and CD137 (also known as Tnfrsf9) [22]. The above-mentioned adipose and beige markers show up-regulation along (see **Figure 1**). The adult thymus expresses PPARgamma, TBX-1 and UCP-1 in the epithelial compartment, and latter two have been reported to initiate beige adipose

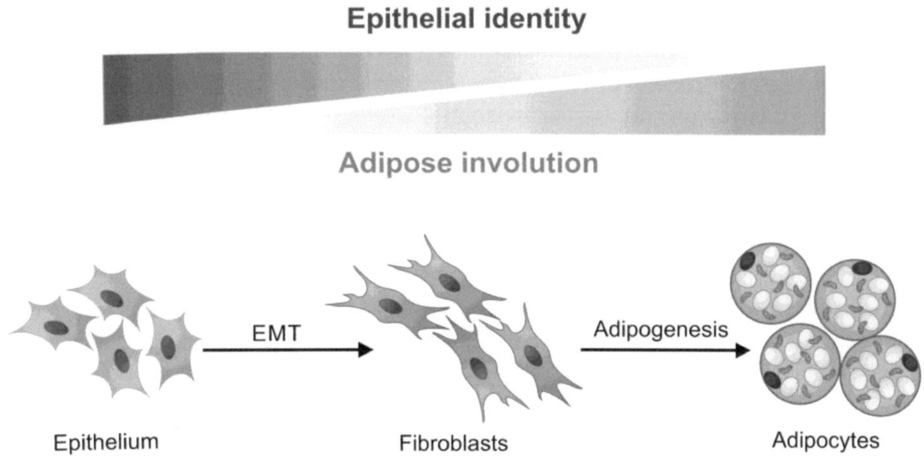

Transcription factors	PPARγ↑, FoxN1↓, TBX1↑
Tissue markers	EpCAM1↓, MHCII↓, Wnt4↓, UCP1↑, CD137↑, EAR2↑
miRNA species	27a↓, 106b↑, 155↓

Figure 1.
Key molecular events of thymic senescence.

tissue development. Thymic adipose tissue may also bee classified based on cellular analysis from an adipocyte perspective [23–26]. Thymus tissue appears to be unique expressing TBX-1 during embryonic development and also during senescence embedded in different contexts. It is appreciable that TBX-1 plays a role in thymus organogenesis (immune peak) and thymic adipose involution (metabolic peak). This suggests an intersection of immunity and metabolism, and a dual role of TBX-1 showing bimodal expression [36].

3. Natural resistance to senescence

A medical condition termed persistent thymus has been known for long [37]. In the affected population the thymus is rescued from involution. These individuals, however, have severe defects in their hormonal system, affecting the level of sex steroids. It is the lack of androgen-effect that prevents thymus involution on one hand, but hampers the endocrine system on the other hand. Recently another medical condition termed FPLD3 (familial partial lipodystrophy type 3) has also been associated with the lack of thymus involution [38]. FPLD3 also derails the hormonal system by affecting PPARgamma activity. As for all adipose tissue subtypes, PPARgamma plays a crucial role during thymus adipose involution as well [39]. It has been suggested by others previously based on direct fate-mapping experiments that with senescence thymic adipose tissue develops from the thymic stromal or epithelial compartment [22]. In further support, epithelial to adipose trans-differentiation has been reported to occur as indicated by the presence by EpCAM-1/PPARgamma double-positive cells at a given time point during thymus senescence. Such cells express cell surface markers as memories of their fading thymic epithelial identity (EpCAM-1), yet already show signs of their novel adipocyte differentiation program in their nuclei (PPARgamma). Further experiments showed that the medullary compartment is rescued from age-related shrinking in case of PPARgamma deficiency. Prolonged survival of thymus stromal niche provides permissive environment for sustained fresh naïve T cell production as indicated by increased mTrec values. Thymocyte subpopulations were equally supported by PPARgamma deficiency and fresh naive T cells outnumbered memory T cells despite age. The sustained support of fresh naive T cells provides functional advantages even at elevated ages. Oral consumption of foreign T-depended antigen initiates immune tolerance to block potential immune response, even along with parallel immunization. Unfortunately, this tolerance is impaired at old age [40–42] Loss of oral tolerance is a potential link to increasing food intolerance prevalence [43–46]. However, tolerance is rescued by PPARgamma deficiency at senior age [38]. In senior individuals protection from seasonal flu strains declines despite annual vaccination [47–49]. The cause: low levels of neutralizing antibody titers due to lacking naïve T-cells required for T-B cooperation. This, however, is also rescued by PPARgamma deficiency [38].

4. Induced rejuvenation

It has been reported early on that the thymus may be regenerated by a variety of interventions (aka thymic rebound) [50]. FoxN1 (a forkhead class transcription factor) is the mastermind of TEC differentiation [51–55]. FoxN1 has also been shown to promote proliferation [56]. Reducing (but not fully diminishing) FoxN1 expression early on triggers premature thymus involution (aka thymus progeria). The opposite, however, over-expression of FoxN1 efficiently postpones thymus involution [57]. Among secreted factors, Wnt4 and keratinocyte growth factor (aka KGF) have also verified as key factors of both thymic senescence and rebound [58–61]. The onset of adolescence presents a frequently proposed physiological cause for thymic degeneration. In accordance, both chemical and surgical castration that result in sex-steroid ablation (SSA) yield thymic rebound [62, 63]. SSA-triggered thymic rebound correlates with both increased thymus size and thymocyte number leading to increased fresh naive T cell production. At the histological level this is suggested by the recovery of the cortico-medullary junction [64]. Accordingly, systemic hormonal changes associated with senescence partly explain changes observed during thymic senescence. In harmony, deletion of the androgen receptor results in an enlarged thymus and resistance to androgen induced thymus atrophy [65]. This is also in line with reports showing that the thymus reaches peak size and productivity early after birth, and not later at puberty [66–68]. Unfortunately, castration-induced rebound is only a transient phenomenon, and the thymus re-involutes within a couple of weeks. Apparently, although SSA may trigger the expansion of the thymus, yet does not rejuvenate it [69]. In the case of the thymus, in comparison with other organs, little is known about the molecular and cellular mechanisms that control its development and maintenance. FoxN1 certainly is a mastermind linking development and maintenance of the thymic microenvironment throughout life, yet some TEC differentiation also occurs independent from Foxn1 [70].

5. Novel trends of rejuvenation

Transcription factor FoxN1 - the mastermind of thymus organogenesis and identity - is a known as the molecular target of the glycolipoprotein Wnt4 [71, 72].

For this reason Wnt4 plays a crucial role in thymus development and maintenance [73–77]. With senescence thymic epithelial cells secrete less Wnt4, however, their Frizzled receptors (Fz4 and Fz6) become up-regulated as compensatory mechanism [78]. It is his loss of Wnt4 expression that allows for thymic adipose involution to develop due to PPARgamma-effect [79, 80]. The Wnt/b-catenin pathway and PPARgamma act as inhibitors of each other hence exogenous Wnt4 can reinforce thymic epithelial identity [79–84]. Wnt4 loses activity when purified, because the Wnt molecules travel in extracellular vesicles (EVs, or exosomes in this case) or on their surfaces [85, 86]. It has been reported that miR27b also specifically inhibits PPARgamma activity [87, 88]. The miRNA species are known travel in EVs and in exosomes as well [89, 90]. The thymus is a rich source of exosomes with immunological relevance in e.g. thymocyte selection [91–94]. As a combination of the above, artificially produced (transgenic) exosomes containing Wnt4 and miR27b in excess can block PPARgamma-effect in thymic epithelial cells thus efficiently counteracting senescence observed as thymic adipose involution [95].

World population is approaching 7.7 billion as of 2019 [96]. Global population increases due to increasing life expectancy, rather than increasing birth rate. However, increasing lifespan is not proportionally attributed with increasing health-span. As a result social expenses rise and novel solutions are urged. Central immune (thymus) senescence research based novel solutions can potentially improve senior immune fitness through decreasing the incidence of infections, malignant and autoimmune disorders. These could also thus alleviate the current burden on healthcare systems and increase quality of life in the elderly. An ultimate goal is to prolong immune fitness and realign it with constantly increasing lifespan.

With aging the thymus shows adipose involution. During this process thymic epithelial cells trans-differentiate into beige adipocytes through an intermediate fibroblast stage. Key molecular events are summarized at the level of transcription factors, tissue markers and miRNA species.

Acknowledgements

The project has been supported by the European Union, cofinanced by the European Social Fund: Comprehensive Development for Implementing Smart Specialization Strategies at the University of Pécs (EFOP-3.6.1.-16-2016-00004).

Author details

Krisztian Kvell
Department of Pharmaceutical Biotechnology, Faculty of Pharmacy, University of Pecs, Pecs, Hungary

*Address all correspondence to: kvell.krisztian@pte.hu

References

[1] Gao S, Li X, Amendt BA. Understanding the role of Tbx1 as a candidate gene for 22q11.2 deletion syndrome. Current Allergy and Asthma Reports. 2013;**13**:613-621. DOI: 10.1007/s11882-013-0384-6

[2] Farley AM, Morris LX, Vroegindeweij E, Depreter MLG, Vaidya H, Stenhouse FH, et al. Dynamics of thymus organogenesis and colonization in early human development. Development. 2013;**140**:2015-2026. DOI: 10.1242/dev.087320

[3] Jerome LA, Papaioannou VE. DiGeorge syndrome phenotype in mice mutant for the T-box gene, Tbx1. Nature Genetics. 2001;**27**:286-291. DOI: 10.1038/85845

[4] Sirianni MC, Businco L, Seminara R, Aiuti F. Severe combined immunodeficiencies, primary T-cell defects and DiGeorge syndrome in humans: Characterization by monoclonal antibodies and natural killer cell activity. Clinical Immunology and Immunopathology. 1983;**28**:361-370. Available at: http://www.ncbi.nlm.nih.gov/pubmed/6349883

[5] Reeh KAG, Cardenas KT, Bain VE, Liu Z, Laurent M, Manley NR, et al. Ectopic TBX1 suppresses thymic epithelial cell differentiation and proliferation during thymus organogenesis. Development. 2014;**141**:2950-2958. DOI: 10.1242/dev.111641

[6] Chinn IK, Blackburn CC, Manley NR, Sempowski GD. Changes in primary lymphoid organs with aging. Seminars in Immunology. 2012;**24**(5):309-320

[7] Chaudhry MS, Velardi E, Dudakov JA, van den Brink MR. Thymus: The next (re)generation. Immunological Reviews. 2016;**271**(1):56-71

[8] Adkins B. T-cell function in newborn mice and humans. Immunology Today. 1999;**20**:330-335

[9] Adkins B. Peripheral CD4+ lymphocytes derived from fetal versus adult thymic precursors differ phenotypically and functionally. Journal of Immunology. 2003;**171**:5157-5164

[10] Min B, McHugh R, Sempowski GD, Mackall C, Foucras G, Paul WE. Neonates support lymphopenia-induced proliferation. Immunity. 2003;**18**:131-140

[11] Anderson G, Jenkinson WE, Jones T, Parnell SM, Kinsella FA, White AJ, et al. Establishment and functioning of intrathymic microenvironments. Immunological Reviews. 2006;**209**:10-27

[12] Gill J, Malin M, Sutherland J, Gray D, Hollander G, Boyd R. Thymic generation and regeneration. Immunological Reviews. 2003;**195**:28-50

[13] Min H, Montecino-Rodriguez E, Dorshkind K. Reduction in the developmental potential of intrathymic T cell progenitors with age. Journal of Immunology. 2004;**173**:245-250

[14] Min H, Montecino-Rodriguez E, Dorshkind K. Reassessing the role of growth hormone and sex steroids in thymic involution. Clinical Immunology. 2006;**118**:117-123

[15] Haynes L, Swain SL. Why aging T cells fail: Implications for vaccination. Immunity. 2006;**24**:663-666

[16] Taub DD, Longo DL. Insights into thymic aging and regeneration. Immunological Reviews. 2005;**205**:72-93

[17] Gray DH, Seach N, Ueno T, Milton MK, Liston A, Lew AM, et al. Developmental kinetics, turnover, and

stimulatory capacity of thymic epithelial cells. Blood. 2006;**108**:3777-3785

[18] Chen L, Xiao S, Manley NR. Foxn1 is required to maintain the postnatal thymic microenvironment in a dosage-sensitive manner. Blood. 2009;**113**:567-574

[19] Griffith AV, Fallahi M, Venables T, Petrie HT. Persistent degenerative changes in thymic organ function revealed by an inducible model of organ regrowth. Aging Cell. 2012;**11**:169-177

[20] Takeoka Y, Chen SY, Yago H, Boyd R, Suehiro S, Shultz LD, et al. The murine thymic microenvironment: Changes with age. International Archives of Allergy and Immunology. 1996;**111**:5-12

[21] Youm YH, Yang H, Amin R, Smith SR, Leff T, Dixit VD. Thiazolidinedione treatment and constitutive-PPARgamma activation induces ectopic adipogenesis and promotes age-related thymic involution. Aging Cell. 2010;**9**:478-489

[22] Youm YH, Yang H, Sun Y, Smith RG, Manley NR, Vandanmagsar B, et al. Deficient ghrelin receptor-mediated signaling compromises thymic stromal cell microenvironment by accelerating thymic adiposity. The Journal of Biological Chemistry. 2009;**284**:7068-7077

[23] Dixit VD. Thymic fatness and approaches to enhance thymopoietic fitness in aging. Current Opinion in Immunology. 2010;**22**:521-528

[24] Sempowski GD, Hale LP, Sundy JS, Massey JM, Koup RA, Douek DC, et al. Leukemia inhibitory factor, oncostatin M, IL-6, and stem cell factor mRNA expression in human thymus increases with age and is associated with thymic atrophy. Journal of Immunology. 2000;**164**:2180-2187

[25] Yang H, Youm YH, Dixit VD. Inhibition of thymic adipogenesis by caloric restriction is coupled with reduction in age-related thymic involution. Journal of Immunology. 2009;**183**:3040-3052

[26] Yang H, Youm YH, Vandanmagsar B, Rood J, Kumar KG, Butler AA, et al. Obesity accelerates thymic aging. Blood. 2009;**114**:3803-3812

[27] Heng TS, Goldberg GL, Gray DH, Sutherland JS, Chidgey AP, Boyd RL. Effects of castration on thymocyte development in two different models of thymic involution. Journal of Immunology. 2005;**175**:2982-2993

[28] Mackall CL, Punt JA, Morgan P, Farr AG, Gress RE. Thymic function in young/old chimeras: Substantial thymic T cell regenerative capacity despite irreversible age-associated thymic involution. European Journal of Immunology. 1998;**28**:1886-1893

[29] Zhu X, Gui J, Dohkan J, Cheng L, Barnes PF, Su DM. Lymphohematopoietic progenitors do not have a synchronized defect with age-related thymic involution. Aging Cell. 2007;**6**:663-672

[30] Klug DB, Crouch E, Carter C, Coghlan L, Conti CJ, Richie ER. Transgenic expression of cyclin D1 in thymic epithelial precursors promotes epithelial and T cell development. Journal of Immunology. 2000;**164**:1881-1888

[31] Nowell CS, Bredenkamp N, Tetelin S, Jin X, Tischner C, Vaidya H, et al. Foxn1 regulates lineage progression in cortical and medullary thymic epithelial cells but is dispensable for medullary sublineage divergence. PLoS Genetics. 2011;**7**:e1002348

[32] Nakayama K, Ishida N, Shirane M, Inomata A, Inoue T, Shishido N, et al. Mice lacking p27(Kip1) display increased body size, multiple organ hyperplasia, retinal dysplasia, and pituitary tumors. Cell. 1996;**85**:707-720

[33] Kiyokawa H, Kineman RD, Manova-Todorova KO, Soares VC, Hoffman ES, Ono M, et al. Enhanced growth of mice lacking the cyclin-dependent kinase inhibitor function of p27(Kip1). Cell. 1996;**85**:721-732

[34] Fero ML, Rivkin M, Tasch M, Porter P, Carow CE, Firpo E, et al. A syndrome of multiorgan hyperplasia with features of gigantism, tumorigenesis, and female sterility in p27(Kip1)-deficient mice. Cell. 1996;**85**:733-744

[35] Sempowski GD, Rhein ME, Scearce RM, Haynes BF. Leukemia inhibitory factor is a mediator of Escherichia coli lipopolysaccharide-induced acute thymic atrophy. European Journal of Immunology. 2002;**32**:3066-3070

[36] Banfai K, Ernszt D, Pap A, Bai P, Garai K, Belharazem D, et al. Beige' cross talk between the immune system and metabolism. Frontiers in Endocrinology. 18 June 2019. https://doi.org/10.3389/fendo.2019.00369

[37] Booth FR. Thymus gland, persistent or overactive. Veterinary Medicine. 1950;**45**(10):387-388

[38] Ernszt D, Banfai K, Kellermayer Z, Pap A, Lord JM, Pongracz JE, et al. PPARgamma deficiency counteracts Thymic senescence. Frontiers in Immunology. 2017;**8**:1515

[39] Kvell K, Varecza Z, Bartis D, Hesse S, Parnell S, Anderson G, et al. Wnt4 and LAP2alpha as pacemakers of thymic epithelial senescence. PLoS One. 2010;**5**(5):e10701

[40] de Faria AM, Ficker SM, Speziali E, Menezes JS, Stransky B, Silva Rodrigues V, et al. Aging affects oral tolerance induction but not its maintenance in mice. Mechanisms of Ageing and Development. 1998;**102**(1):67-80

[41] Kato H, Fujihashi K, Kato R, Dohi T, Fujihashi K, Hagiwara Y, et al. Lack of oral tolerance in aging is due to sequential loss of Peyer's patch cell interactions. International Immunology. 2003;**15**(2):145-158

[42] Song F, Guan Z, Gienapp IE, Shawler T, Benson J, Whitacre CC. The thymus plays a role in oral tolerance in experimental autoimmune encephalomyelitis. Journal of Immunology. 2006;**177**(3):1500-1509

[43] Galipeau HJ, Verdu EF. Gut microbes and adverse food reactions: Focus on gluten related disorders. Gut Microbes. 2014;**5**(5):594-605. DOI: 10.4161/19490976.2014.969635

[44] Marietta EV, Murray JA. Animal models to study gluten sensitivity. Seminars in Immunopathology. 2012;**34**(4):497-511. DOI: 10.1007/s00281-012-0315-y

[45] MacDonald TT. Evidence for cell-mediated hypersensitivity as an important pathogenetic mechanism in food intolerance. Clinical and Experimental Allergy. 1995;**25**(Suppl 1):10-13

[46] Ferguson A, Ziegler K, Strobel S. Gluten intolerance (coeliac disease). Annals of Allergy. 1984;**53**(6 Pt 2):637-642

[47] Cromer D, van Hoek AJ, Jit M, Edmunds WJ, Fleming D, Miller E. The burden of influenza in England by age and clinical risk group: A statistical analysis to inform vaccine policy. The Journal of Infection. 2014;**68**(4):363-371. DOI: 10.1016/j.jinf.2013.11.013

[48] Ang LW, Lim C, Lee VJ, Ma S, Tiong WW, Ooi PL, et al. Influenza-associated hospitalizations, Singapore, 2004-2008 and 2010-2012. Emerging Infectious Diseases. 2014;**20**(10):1652-1660. DOI: 10.3201/eid2010.131768

[49] Haq K, McElhaney JE. Immunosenescence: Influenza vaccination and the elderly. Current Opinion in Immunology. 2014;**29**:38-42. DOI: 10.1016/j.coi.2014.03.008

[50] Billard MJ, Gruver AL, Sempowski GD. Acute endotoxin-induced Thymic atrophy is characterized by intrathymic inflammatory and wound healing responses. PLoS One. 2011;**6**:e17940

[51] Hale JS, Boursalian TE, Turk GL, Fink PJ. Thymic output in aged mice. Proceedings of the National Academy of Sciences of the United States of America. 2006;**103**:8447-8452

[52] Kaestner KH, Knochel W, Martinez DE. Unified nomenclature for the winged helix/forkhead transcription factors. Genes & Development. 2000;**14**:142-146

[53] Nehls M, Pfeifer D, Schorpp M, Hedrich H, Boehm T. New member of the winged-helix protein family disrupted in mouse and rat nude mutations. Nature. 1994;**372**:103-107

[54] Nehls M, Kyewski B, Messerle M, Waldschütz R, Schüddekopf K, Smith AJ, et al. Two genetically separable steps in the differentiation of thymic epithelium. Science. 1996;**272**:886-889

[55] Blackburn CC, Augustine CL, Li R, Harvey RP, Malin MA, Boyd RL, et al. The nu gene acts cell-autonomously and is required for differentiation of thymic epithelial progenitors. Proceedings of the National Academy of Sciences of the United States of America. 1996;**93**:5742-5746

[56] Su DM, Navarre S, Oh WJ, Condie BG, Manley NR. A domain of Foxn1 required for crosstalkdependent thymic epithelial cell differentiation. Nature Immunology. 2003;**4**:1128-1135

[57] Itoi M, Kawamoto H, Katsura Y, Amagai T. Two distinct steps of immigration of hematopoietic progenitors into the early thymus anlage. International Immunology. 2001;**13**:1203-1211

[58] Zook EC, Krishack PA, Zhang S, Zeleznik-Le NJ, Firulli AB, Witte PL, et al. Overexpression of Foxn1 attenuates age-associated thymic involution and prevents the expansion of peripheral CD4 memory T cells. Blood. 2011

[59] Suniara RK, Jenkinson EJ, Owen JJ. An essential role for thymic mesenchyme in early T cell development. The Journal of Experimental Medicine. 2000;**191**:1051-1056

[60] Erickson M, Morkowski S, Lehar S, Gillard G, Beers C, Dooley J, et al. Regulation of thymic epithelium by keratinocyte growth factor. Blood. 2002;**100**:3269-3278

[61] Revest JM, Suniara RK, Kerr K, Owen JJ, Dickson C. Development of the thymus requires signaling through the fibroblast growth factor receptor r2-iiib. Journal of Immunology. 2001;**167**:1954-1961

[62] Rossi SW, Jeker LT, Ueno T, Kuse S, Keller MP, Zuklys S, et al. Keratinocyte growth factor (KGF) enhances postnatal T-cell development via enhancements in proliferation and function of thymic epithelial cells. Blood. 2007;**109**:3803-3811

[63] Fitzpatrick FT, Kendall MD, Wheeler MJ, Adcock IM, Greenstein BD. Reappearance of thymus of ageing rats after orchidectomy. The Journal of Endocrinology. 1985;**106**:R17-R19

[64] Hince M, Sakkal S, Vlahos K, Dudakov J, Boyd R, Chidgey A. The role of sex steroids and gonadectomy in the control of thymic involution. Cellular Immunology. 2008;**252**:122-138

[65] Olsen NJ, Olson G, Viselli SM, Gu X, Kovacs WJ. Androgen receptors in thymic epithelium modulate thymus size and thymocyte development. Endocrinology. 2001;**142**:1278-1283

[66] Steinmann GG. Changes in the human thymus during aging. Current Topics in Pathology. 1986;**75**:43-88

[67] Steinmann GG, Klaus B, Muller-Hermelink HK. The involution of the ageing human thymic epithelium is independent of puberty. A morphometric study. Scandinavian Journal of Immunology. 1985;**22**:563-575

[68] George AJ, Ritter MA. Thymic involution with ageing: Obsolescence or good housekeeping? Immunology Today. 1996;**17**:267-272

[69] Henderson J. On the relationship of the thymus to the sexual organs. Journal of Physiology. 1904;**31**:222-229

[70] Zamisch M, Moore-Scott B, Su DM, Lucas PJ, Manley N, Richie ER. Ontogeny and regulation of IL-7-expressing thymic epithelial cells. Journal of Immunology. 2005;**174**:60-67

[71] Romano R, Palamaro L, Fusco A, Giardino G, Gallo V, Del Vecchio L, et al. FOXN1: A master regulator gene of Thymic epithelial development program. Frontiers in Immunology. 2013;**4**:187. DOI: 10.3389/fimmu.2013.00187

[72] Kvell K, Varecza Z, Bartis D, Hesse S, Parnell S, Anderson G, et al. Wnt4 and LAP2alpha as pacemakers of thymic epithelial senescence. PLoS One. 2010;**5**:e10701. DOI: 10.1371/journal.pone.0010701

[73] Pongracz JE, Parnell SM, Jones T, Anderson G, Jenkinson EJ. Overexpression of ICAT highlights a role for catenin-mediated canonical Wnt signalling in early T cell development. European Journal of Immunology. 2006;**36**:2376-2383. DOI: 10.1002/eji.200535721

[74] Kvell K, Fejes AV, Parnell SM, Pongracz JE. Active Wnt/beta-catenin signaling is required for embryonic thymic epithelial development and functionality ex vivo. Immunobiology. 2014;**219**:644-652. DOI: 10.1016/j.imbio.2014.03.017

[75] Heinonen KM, Vanegas JR, Brochu S, Shan J, Vainio SJ, Perreault C. Wnt4 regulates thymic cellularity through the expansion of thymic epithelial cells and early thymic progenitors. Blood. 2011;**118**:5163-5173. DOI: 10.1182/blood-2011-04-350553

[76] Taub DD, Longo DL. Insights into thymic aging and regeneration. Immunological Reviews. 2005;**205**:72-93. DOI: 10.1111/j.0105-2896.2005.00275.x

[77] Pongracz J, Hare K, Harman B, Anderson G, Jenkinson EJ. Thymic epithelial cells provide Wnt signals to developing thymocytes. European Journal of Immunology. 2003;**33**:1949-1956. DOI: 10.1002/eji.200323564

[78] Varecza Z, Kvell K, Talabér G, Miskei G, Csongei V, Bartis D, et al. Multiple suppression pathways of canonical Wnt signalling control thymic epithelial senescence. Mechanisms of Ageing and Development. 2011;**132**:249-256. DOI: 10.1016/j.mad.2011.04.007

[79] Marinova TT. Epithelial framework reorganization during human thymus involution. Gerontology. 2005;**51**:14-18. DOI: 10.1159/000081429

[80] Talaber G, Kvell K, Varecza Z, Boldizsar F, Parnell SM, Jenkinson EJ, et al. Wnt-4 protects thymic epithelial cells against dexamethasone-induced senescence. Rejuvenation Research. 2011;**14**:241-248. DOI: 10.1089/rej.2010.1110

[81] Gustafson B, Smith U. The WNT inhibitor Dickkopf 1 and bone morphogenetic protein 4 rescue adipogenesis in hypertrophic obesity in humans. Diabetes. 2012;**61**:1217-1224. DOI: 10.2337/db11-1419

[82] Lecarpentier Y, Claes V, Vallée A, Hébert J-L. Thermodynamics in cancers: Opposing interactions between PPAR gamma and the canonical WNT/beta-catenin pathway. Clinical and Translational Medicine. 2017;**6**:14. DOI: 10.1186/s40169-017-0144-7

[83] Lecarpentier Y, Vallée A. Opposite interplay between PPAR gamma and canonical Wnt/Beta-catenin pathway in amyotrophic lateral sclerosis. Frontiers in Neurology. 2016;7:100. DOI: 10.3389/fneur.2016.00100

[84] Kvell K, Pongracz JE. Central Immune Senescence, Reversal Potentials. Rijeka: InTech; 2012. Available at: http://www.ncbi.nlm.nih.gov/pubmed/28045481 [Accessed: 04-July-2018]

[85] Willert K, Brown JD, Danenberg E, Duncan AW, Weissman IL, Reya T, et al. Wnt proteins are lipid-modified and can act as stem cell growth factors. Nature. 2003;**423**:448-452. DOI: 10.1038/nature01611

[86] Zhang L, Wrana JL. The emerging role of exosomes in Wnt secretion and transport. Current Opinion in Genetics & Development. 2014;**27**:14-19. DOI: 10.1016/j.gde.2014.03.006

[87] Wang T, Xu Z. miR-27 promotes osteoblast differentiation by modulating Wnt signaling. Biochemical and Biophysical Research Communications. 2010;**402**:186-189. DOI: 10.1016/j.bbrc.2010.08.031

[88] Jennewein C, von Knethen A, Schmid T, Brüne B. MicroRNA-27b contributes to lipopolysaccharide-mediated peroxisome proliferator-activated receptor gamma (PPARgamma) mRNA destabilization. The Journal of Biological Chemistry. 2010;**285**:11846-11853. DOI: 10.1074/jbc.M109.066399

[89] Gross JC, Chaudhary V, Bartscherer K, Boutros M. Active Wnt proteins are secreted on exosomes. Nature Cell Biology. 2012;**14**:1036-1045. DOI: 10.1038/ncb2574

[90] Xu D, Tahara H. The role of exosomes and microRNAs in senescence and aging. Advanced Drug Delivery Reviews. 2013;**65**:368-375. DOI: 10.1016/j.addr.2012.07.010

[91] Skogberg G, Telemo E, Ekwall O. Exosomes in the thymus: Antigen transfer and vesicles. Frontiers in Immunology. 2015;**6**:366. DOI: 10.3389/fimmu.2015.00366

[92] Turiák L, Misják P, Szabó TG, Aradi B, Pálóczi K, Ozohanics O, et al. Proteomic characterization of thymocyte-derived microvesicles and apoptotic bodies in BALB/c mice. Journal of Proteomics. 2011;**74**:2025-2033. DOI: 10.1016/j.jprot.2011.05.023

[93] Skogberg G, Gudmundsdottir J, van der Post S, Sandström K, Bruhn S, Benson M, et al. Characterization of human thymic exosomes. PLoS One. 2013;**8**:e67554. DOI: 10.1371/journal.pone.0067554

[94] Lundberg V, Berglund M, Skogberg G, Lindgren S, Lundqvist C, Gudmundsdottir J, et al. Thymic exosomes promote the final maturation of thymocytes. Scientific Reports. 2016;**6**:36479. DOI: 10.1038/srep36479

[95] Banfai K, Garai K, Ernszt D, Pongracz JE, Kvell K. Transgenic exosomes for thymus regeneration. Frontiers in Immunology. 2019;**10**:862. DOI: 10.3389/fimmu.2019.00862

[96] Available from: https://population.io/

Chapter 5

Age-Related Thymic Atrophy: Mechanisms and Outcomes

Rachel Thomas and Dong-Ming Su

Abstract

Age-related thymic atrophy or involution, a hallmark of thymic aging, takes place both in humans and animals. In this chapter, we will discuss age-related thymic atrophy, outlining the underlying cellular and molecular mechanisms of its occurrence. We will also address the downstream influences on the aged T cell immune system, not only regarding insufficiency against pathogens, but also hyper-reactivity to self. Particularly, we will focus on how thymic atrophy disrupts efficient establishment of central T cell immune tolerance primarily via impairment of thymocyte negative selection, resulting in an increased number of self-reactive conventional T cells, and on thymic-derived regulatory T cell generation. Finally, we will provide a framework for understanding the significant role that the atrophied thymus plays in shaping inflammaging: a chronic, low-grade, systemic inflammatory phenotype observed in aged individuals in the absence of acute infection. The involvement of T cell adaptive immunity in mediating inflammaging plays a crucial role in the progression of many age-related neurological and cardiovascular diseases.

Keywords: thymic atrophy, aging, inflammaging, central tolerance, regulatory T (Treg) cells

1. Introduction

The thymus gland is the primary central lymphoid organ involved in development and selection of T lymphocytes (T cells) [1]. It is also responsible for the establishment of central T cell immune tolerance, which includes two mechanisms: thymocyte negative selection, through which most self (auto)-reactive T cells are depleted [2], and the generation of CD4 single positive ($CD4^{SP}$)$FoxP3^{+}$ regulatory T (Treg) cells [3], which act to suppress self-reactive T cell-mediated reactions in the periphery [4]. It is thought that Treg cells provide some level of compensation for imperfections in negative selection that allow some self-reactive T cells to escape this protective process [5]. As part of the aging process, the thymus undergoes progressive involution or atrophy in most vertebrates, exhibiting not only morphological changes, but also a functional decline resulting in [6, 7] significantly lowered thymic output [8].

The theoretical causes of this age-related diminishment of thymopoiesis are two-fold. First, is the notion of a hematopoietic defect. This stems from the observations that there are reduced numbers of hematopoietic stem cell (HSC) progenitors produced by the bone marrow with age, [9] that could cause a reduction in early T-cell progenitors (ETP) entering the thymus [10]. Second, is the notion of a non-hematopoietic defect, which suggests that the primary age-related atrophy of the thymus is derived from HSC niche cells [11, 12] and thymic stromal cells, or ETP niches [13, 14]. The myriad of changes that characterize thymic atrophy first occur within the thymic niche and then extend to the ETPs as a result of age. We believe that these substantial age-related alterations in thymic microstructure and microenvironment, which provide important thymic factors, contribute more heavily to the diminished thymopoiesis observed in the elderly [7, 13] The primary thymic stromal cells are thymic epithelial cells (TECs), including two subpopulations distinct in their localization, function, and molecular expression patterns, namely medullary TECs (mTECs) and cortical TECs (cTECs) [15]. Compelling evidence show that age-related thymic atrophy is tightly associated with postnatal TEC homeostasis, which is regulated by TEC autonomous transcription factors (TFs), such as Forkhead box N1 (FoxN1) [16].

Age-related changes to immune system function, often referred to as immunosenescence [17–20], are generally thought of as immune insufficiency, such as reduced anti-infection and vaccine immunity [21] and reduced tumor surveillance [22, 23]. However, self-reactive immune responses are elevated in the elderly, which is a result of inflammaging, a chronic, low-grade, systemic inflammatory phenotype in the absence of acute infection observed in aged individuals [24–31]. Immunosenescence and inflammaging are antagonistic phenotypes, but they actually comprise two sides of the same coin in terms of age-related immune dysregulation [19, 20, 32, 33]. It has been proposed that the basal inflammatory state defined by inflammaging greatly contributes to many age-related degenerative diseases, including neurodegenerative diseases, such as Alzheimer's disease, metabolic diseases, and cardiovascular diseases, among others [30, 34, 35].

Here, we will outline the cellular and molecular mechanisms underlying the occurrence of age-related thymic atrophy including some of the aforementioned hallmarks, and its effects on general T cell output. We will also describe its effects on the establishment of central T cell immune tolerance via a combination of both mechanistic arms of central tolerance: thymocyte negative selection and thymic-derived $CD4^{SP}FoxP3^{+}$ T regulatory (tTreg) cell generation. We will discuss why we believe many aspects of the adaptive immune system's role in the development of inflammaging can be attributed to these thymic manifestations. Finally, in light of new trends in T cell immune system aging, we will expand on some future research goals in the field of thymic atrophy interventions and therapeutics as a potential conduit for normalizing aged T cell-mediated immunity. This is of clinical significance for combating age-related neurological and cardiovascular diseases.

2. Hallmarks of age-related thymic atrophy

During aging, the thymus undergoes progressive atrophy [36]. In addition to a reduction in thymic mass (size and thymocyte numbers), there is substantial remodeling of the thymic microstructure. The thymus is characterized by two primary compartments, namely the cortex and the medulla. In between the cortex and medulla, there is a zone termed the corticomedullary junction (CMJ) (**Figure 1a**). These two compartments contain specialized thymic epithelial cells (TECs), cortical (cTECs) or medullary (mTECs), and these cellular compartments are responsible for different stages of thymocyte development and selection [37, 38]. Regarding thymic microstructure, the aged, involuted thymus, in addition to an overall decline in TEC-associated markers, such as keratin and major histocompatibility complex class-II (MHC-II), also manifests altered ratios of cTECs to mTECs, and an overt change in microstructure due to disrupted

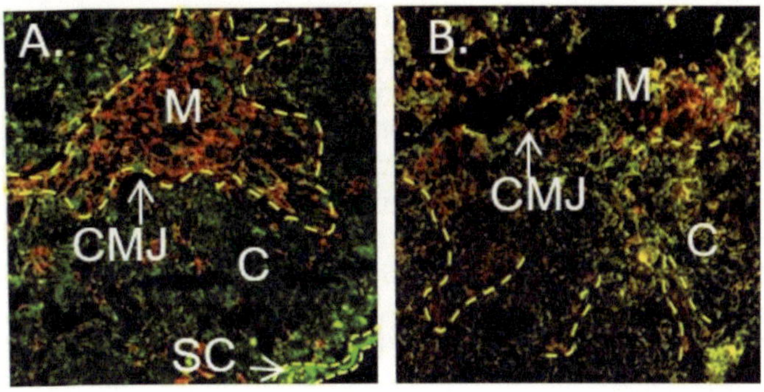

Figure 1.
Thymic microstructural changes characterized by K8 and K5 fluorescent staining. In the aged thymus, the CMJ is not clear, because the medulla is disorganized and medullary TECs are dispersed and do not form a distinct compartmental region. Normally, $K8^+$ TECs (green) are primarily localized in the cortical region, while $K5^+$ TECs (red) are primarily localized in the medullary region. A) Young (~2 months old) murine thymus; B) aged (>18 months old) murine thymus. C = cortex, M = medulla, CMJ = corticomedullary junction, SC = subcapsule.

CMJ, resulting in a disorganized medullary region (**Figure 1b**). A decline in MHC-II^{hi} expressing TECs is a sign of the reduction of mature mTECs [39, 40]. Additionally, increased numbers of fibroblasts [39] and accumulation of adipose tissue in the thymus is also observed [40].

Increased senescent cells (β-Gal^+, $p21^+$, and $TAP63^+$) [41] in the aged thymus are also present, and it has been demonstrated that TECs contribute to the senescence observed in the aged thymus [39, 41, 42]. This possibly contributes to an increased inflammatory environment (increased levels of IL-6, IL-1β, etc.) within the involuted thymus [30, 43]. Additionally, there is augmented apoptosis in TECs of the atrophied thymus, contributing to diminished stromal cellularity [39].

3. Mechanisms of age-related thymic atrophy

3.1 Mechanisms of diminished thymic input and output associated with aged thymus

Perhaps the most noted outcome of age-related thymic atrophy is diminished thymic output and thymopoesis. This attracts attention and has led many groups to examine whether the bone marrow (BM) derived hematopoietic stem cell (HSC) lymphoid progenitors are sufficiently able to seed the thymus during aging. This is because HSCs are reduced [9] with a myeloid biased development in advanced age [44]. There have been many studies investigating this aspect of thymopoiesis and it is suggested that age-related HSCs contain defects [9] that could contribute to insufficient entry of early T-cell progenitors (ETPs) into the aged thymus [10]. Thus, this result could explain decreased thymic output with age [45].

Mechanisms of diminished thymic input resulting in thymic involution and declined thymic output are mainly based on bone marrow transplantation (BMT) experiments using mouse models. In these models, transferring aged HSCs into young mice could not rejuvenate the thymic involution induced by irradiation prior to bone marrow transplantation [46]. Additionally, the HSC progenitors have been shown to exhibit an age-related skewed proportion within the HSC pool towards myeloid lineage versus lymphoid lineage [44, 47–49]. It has also been observed that early stage thymocytes, defined as the ETPs in the triple negative-1 (TN1) thymocyte population, from aged mice demonstrated decreased differentiation after *in vitro* fetal thymic organ culture [10]. This group also reported declined proliferation and enhanced apoptosis of these early thymocytes taken from aged animals compared to young controls. The overall assertion was that the deficiency in thymocyte differentiation and development past this early stage was attributed to the production of the HSCs in the aged bone marrow [10]. Therefore, aged HSCs and ETPs were regarded as having an intrinsic defect [50].

Given the comprehensive microenvironments in young and aged animals, and the vulnerability of HSCs or ETPs during *in vitro* preparation, these experiments using BMT and ETP culture may not provide the necessary rigor for the conclusions drawn from them, and certainly do not adequately reflect physiological conditions. Therefore, we designed an age-mismatched experimental system with less *in vitro* preparation to reexamine these biological events [13, 51]. One design was to utilize young or aged IL-7R knockout mice as recipients [13, 52, 53], in which their BM niche is relatively open and available to accept exogenous BM cells without irradiation [52, 54]. After grafting young BM cells into young and aged IL-7R knockout mice, the young BM cells produced a young profile in young recipients, but the same young BM cells produced an old profile in aged recipients [13], which implies that the microenvironment directs BM cell aging, rather than the HSCs themselves [14]. The other design was to utilize mouse fetal thymus transplantation into young or aged mice, in which BM progenitors from young or aged recipients seed the grafted young thymus *in vivo* [51]. After grafting fetal thymic lobes into young and aged wild-type recipient mice, BM progenitors from young and old mice were able to grow equally well in the engrafted thymus (with young thymic microenvironment) [51]. In addition, aged HSCs seeding the engrafted thymus did not demonstrate any intrinsic defects [13, 55]. These comprehensive experiments provide solid evidence that the non-hematopoietic microenvironment, rather than HSCs, direct hematopoietic progenitor aging [14], thereby mediating the kinetics of thymic involution [7].

An important fact linking these potential mechanisms is the unique cross-talk or interaction that occurs between the developing hematopoietic progenitors (such as thymocytes) and the stromal microenvironment (such as TECs) in the thymus [15]. For example, there are reports that several key thymic factors involved in this cross-talk are adversely impacted by age-related thymic atrophy. One such factor is IL-7, secreted by TECs, which is important for thymopoiesis and has been shown to be reduced in the aged thymus [56]. Interestingly, direct exogenous supplementation of IL-7 helped to improve aged thymopoiesis [57]. On the other hand, thymocytes provide signals to promote TEC development, at least during thymic organogenesis [58, 59], but the dynamics of this phenomenon during thymic aging remain unknown.

In general, adult organ size is governed by the tissue-specific stem cell pool [60, 61]. It is known that there are two types of tissue-specific stem pools: infinite pools, such as in the liver, and restricted pools, such as in the pancreas. For example, if the liver is injured, its infinite stem pool can expand at a high capacity; whereas, if the pancreas is injured, the expansion of its tissue-specific stem cell pool is very limited due to its restricted and finite epithelial progenitor pool. The thymic epithelial progenitor pool has characteristics of the restricted, finite epithelial progenitor pool [61]. Therefore, it is conceivable that aging TECs exhibit limited turnover compared to mobile thymocytes, which are periodically entering from the BM [62, 63].

Taken together, deficiencies in thymocyte-TEC interactions in the thymus [15] promote thymic atrophy during aging. However, given the fact that thymocytes are mobile with a relatively short period of thymic residency, while TECs have permanent residency in the thymus, experimental evidence [13, 51] and the "seed and soil" theory describing how the soil (stem niche) directs seed (HSC) fate [64–66], lead us to conclude that age-related thymic involution begins with defects in the TEC compartment.

3.2 Mechanisms of thymic stromal cell-mediated structural thymic atrophy

In light of the aforementioned evidence of age-related TEC defects and the decline in total TEC numbers in the aged, atrophied thymus, we now move to discuss the underlying mechanisms of these alterations. Many studies have been conducted to identify factors involved in the cellular and molecular aspects of TEC aging (cytokines, transcription factors, microRNAs, sex steroids, etc.). The single most predominant factor currently accepted as significantly contributing to this phenomenon is the TEC autonomous transcription factor FoxN1. This idea was based on the athymic nude mouse phenotype [67, 68]. FoxN1 is expressed mainly in epithelial cells of the thymus and skin to regulate epithelial cell differentiation in these organs [67]. It is thereby responsible for thymic organogenesis and subsequent T cell development in the thymus [16], as well as hair follicle development in the skin [69, 70]. Many past and current studies utilize nude mice, which exhibit a null mutation in FoxN1 resulting in the lack of hair and the thymus, which explains the lack of T cells in these mice [71, 72].

FoxN1 is noted to be reduced in expression in the age-related atrophied thymus and has even been described as one of the first markers of the onset of thymic involution [73, 74]. The question is whether this reduced FoxN1 expression is due to TEC aging, which results in a decline in many TEC-associated genes, or if primary FoxN1 decline with aging induces a TEC defect that then results in age-related thymic involution. This cause-and-effect relationship had been substantially debated prior to the generation of a conditional knock-out (cKO) FoxN1 mouse model [75]. In this model, the murine FoxN1 gene is *loxP*-floxed and the $uCreER^{T}$ is introduced through crossbreeding [76]. In this model, the tamoxifen (TM)-inducible ubiquitous Cre-recombinase ($uCreER^{T}$) transgene has a low level of spontaneous activation, even without TM induction [77, 78], causing gradual excision of the $FoxN1^{flox/flox}$ gene over time. This results in progressive loss of FoxN1 with age and thymic involution that is positively correlated with reduced FoxN1 levels [79]. Supplying exogenous FoxN1, such as via plasmid [79] or transgene [80, 81], into the aged thymus greatly reduces thymic atrophy and improves function. Additionally, the use of FoxN1 reporter mice has enabled further elucidation of the timeline and kinetics of thymic atrophy with age [82]. For example, one group recently published a study demonstrating that the reduction in FoxN1 initiates the onset of thymic involution, beginning predominantly in the cTEC compartment [82]. Therefore, a decline in FoxN1 expression with aging causally induces flaws in TEC homeostasis, thereby resulting in age-related thymic atrophy, as opposed to the notion that age-induced thymic atrophy causes FoxN1 decline in the thymus.

4. Outcomes of age-related thymic atrophy

Overt outcomes of age-related thymic atrophy include reduction of functional naïve T cells, which is related to a decline in T cell receptor (TCR) repertoire diversity [8, 55, 83, 84]. However, the atrophied thymus is still functioning, albeit with limitations, in the elderly, continuing to select T cells for the lifetime of the individual. This causes a potential for the atrophied thymus to generate harmful T cells that could increase autoimmune predisposition the elderly [26]. Therefore, we will review recent research progress regarding this area of concern.

4.1 Decreased naïve conventional T cell output

As stated previously, the most readily observed outcome of age-related thymic involution is the decline in thymic output, which includes reduced naïve conventional T (Tcon) cell output over time [85] and fewer recent thymic emigrants (RTEs) [8]. However, peripheral T cell numbers are not decreased in aged individuals [36, 86, 87]. The actual effect is an overall diminished TCR repertoire diversity observed in the aged peripheral T cell pool [8, 55, 83, 84], which is due to oligoclonal expansion of memory T cells along with insufficient RTE output. This has been suggested to contribute to the decreased capacity for new immune responses to infection and poor vaccination efficacy, which are typical phenotypes of immunosenescence [17–20], observed in the elderly [35].

This phenotype has been recapitulated in FoxN1 cKO mice, which have accelerated aging in the thymus, but maintain a young periphery, as they exhibit impaired peripheral T cell responses in infection with influenza virus [88]. This study also demonstrated a direct role for thymic atrophy in the impairment of T cell function during aging.

4.2 Increased self-reactive conventional T cells due to perturbed negative selection

In light of the alterations in thymocyte number and diminished naïve T cell output with age-related thymic atrophy, it is of paramount importance to understand the effects of the altered thymic micro-environment on central tolerance establishment of the thymocytes that are still being developed in the atrophied thymus.

Under the current paradigm, negative selection is the process by which thymocytes with high affinity for self-peptides presented by MHC are deleted from the developing thymocyte repertoire via apoptosis [2, 38, 89]. Studies also show that when these high affinity TCRs receive strong signaling, negative selection takes place [90, 91]. However, the TCR signaling strength is not based solely on TCR affinity, but is also influenced by avidity, or the quantity of interactions between self-peptide/MHC (self-pMHC) complexes and the TCR (**Figure 2**). Therefore, if the thymocyte-intrinsic factors (i.e., TCR affinity and number), of self-reactive thymocytes are unchanged, the TCR signaling strength varies based on the ability of effective self-pMHC-II expression. In other words, if self-antigen can be normally presented in the MHC-II groove, the reciprocal TCR signaling should be produced through a strong interaction. We know that MHC-II is expressed on mTECs, however, aging induces mTEC defects (**Figure 1b**), resulting in reduced capacity for self-pMHC-II ligand expression. Therefore, we suggest that a strong signaling strength shifts either to an intermediate strength, which favors $CD4^{SP}FoxP3^{+}$ tTreg cell generation (**Figure 2**, arrow-a), or to a low strength, which results in the generation of self-reactive thymocytes (**Figure 2**, arrow-b). The self-reactive thymocytes via this pathway are neither depleted nor shifted to Treg cells, but become Tcon cells that are released to the periphery. If they encounter specific self-tissues, they may become effector T (Teff) cells that can attack self-tissues and induce pathological inflammation.

The FoxN1 cKO mouse model is a useful model for studying the capacity for efficient self-pMHC-II ligand expression, because it exhibits a defect in the non-hematopoietic TECs, but maintains intrinsically normal hematopoietic lineage cells and a young periphery. We demonstrated that thymic involution perturbs negative selection, as revealed by the enhanced release of autoreactive interphotoreceptor retinoid-binding protein (IRBP)-specific Tcon cells from the atrophied thymus of FoxN1 cKO mice compared to the thymus from young normal controls [25]. This

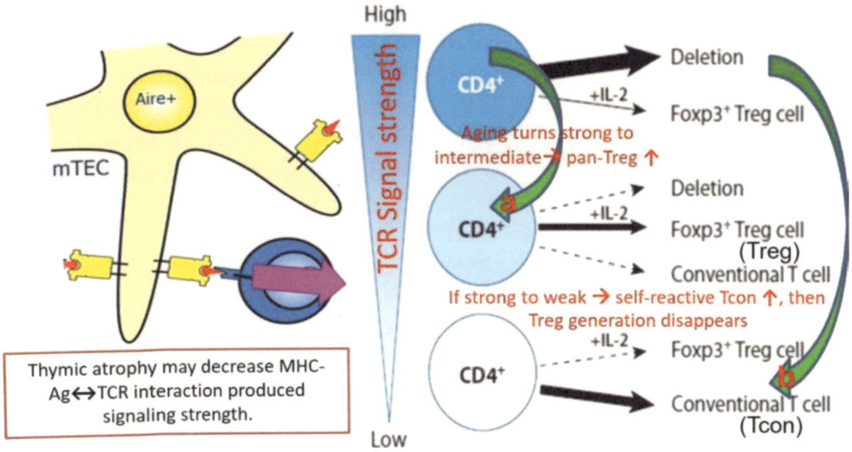

Figure 2.
Signaling strength decides self-reactive CD4^{SP} T clone fates. Interaction between self-pMHC on mTEC and self-reactive TCR on CD4^{SP} thymocyte produces thress types of signaling strength: a strong signal leads to negative selection, resulting in depletion, an intermediate signal leads to tTreg generation, and a weak signal results in thymocyte survival to differentiate into Tcon. Thymic aging (green arrow—a) shifts signaling strength from strong to intermediate and relatively enhances polyclonal tTreg generation; while some antigen-specific interactions exhibit an extremely weak signal, resulting in diminished antigen-specific tTreg cells and increased antigen-specific Tcon cells (green arrow—b).

result is presumably due to decreased self-pMHC-II expression, confirmed via assessment of a mock self-antigen in normal versus atrophied thymus [92].

4.3 Changes in thymic-derived regulatory T cell generation

As mentioned earlier, central tolerance establishment encompasses two mechanisms. The first mechanism, negative selection, is not entirely perfect [5] resulting in some self-reactive T clones being released into the periphery as Tcon cells. The second defense against self-reactivity is CD4^{SP}FoxP3^{+} peripheral Treg (pTreg) cell-mediated autoimmune suppression. It is believed that 80–95% of pTreg cells are generated within the thymus, as thymic-derived T regulatory (tTreg) cells [93–95]. Under the current paradigm, the processes of both negative selection and tTreg generation in the thymus utilize the same set of agonist self-peptides [93, 96]. Whether self-reactive thymocytes developing in the thymus are negatively selected or develop into tTreg cells depends on TCR signaling strength, or the sum of TCR affinity and avidity, (or the number of TCR interactions with self-peptide/MHC) when all other variables, such as IL-2, etc., are fixed. Put simply, strong signaling induces the apoptosis of self-reactive thymocytes, intermediate signaling leads to tTreg generation, and weak signaling results in the survival of thymocytes that differentiate into Tcon cells (**Figure 2**). This paradigm implies that depletion or survival for thymocytes is dependent on overall TCR signaling strength [38, 93].

Although there are cell extrinsic factors that can impact thymocyte development, such as the thymic cytokine milieu (IL-2 [97, 98], TGF-β [98, 99], etc.), we propose that there are two cell types that directly regulate TCR signaling strength. One is intrinsic to thymocytes and the other is intrinsic to TECs. When the TCR binds to self-peptide/MHC on an antigen presenting cell, the immunoreceptor tyrosine-based activation motifs (ITAMs) are activated and the Zap70 kinase is subsequently phosphorylated. A mouse model with a knock-in allele of TCR zeta (ζ) chain gene with tyrosine-to-phenylalanine mutations in 6 out of 10 ITAMs led to a 60% decrease in TCR signaling potential [100]. This mouse model exhibited a defect in negative selection, but an increase in tTreg generation [100]. The second variable is the relative expression level of self-peptide/MHC on TECs. Transgenic expression of a microRNA targeting the MHC class-II transactivator (CIITA) resulted in reduced MHC-II on mTECs [37], leading to insufficient mTEC presentation of self-peptides thus reducing the overall avidity of the TCR interaction with self-peptide/MHC. This also resulted in the enhancement of tTreg generation at the expense of negative selection [37].

In the aged thymus, as we mentioned earlier, mTECs are flawed and self-antigen cannot be normally presented in the MHC-II groove, which results in a diminished interaction with TCRs on developing thymocytes. This is similar to the second scenario described above, in which a defect exists in the TEC compartment causing reduced TCR signaling strength. We observed a relatively enhanced tTreg generation in the atrophied thymus, exhibiting no change in overall tTreg numbers, but an increased ratio of tTreg to tTcon cells in the aged, atrophied thymus compared to young controls [92]. This is probably a demonstration of the atrophied thymus attempting to compensate for defective negative selection [25] in order to maintain central T cell tolerance in the elderly.

If self-reactive TCR signaling strength is too low these thymocytes may neither be depleted nor form tTreg cells, but rather may directly differentiate into self-reactive Tcon cells. As an artifact of impaired promiscuous self-antigen expression in mTECs through an autoimmune regulator (*Aire*) knock-out model, the *Aire*-dependent TCAF3 epitope of prostate antigen cannot be promiscuously expressed on mTECs [101]. This resulted in prostate-specific thymocytes, which should be negatively selected, but in contrast were redirected into prostate-reactive Tcon cells. The authors observed loss of prostate-specific tTreg cells for this same epitope, and heightened prostate-reactive Tcon cells that infiltrated the prostate of these mice causing auto-inflammatory lesions [102, 103]. Defects in self-peptide expression on mTECs due to protein knock-out [104], are beginning to suggest that some of the same impairments exhibited by the atrophied thymus, may impact antigen-specific (monoclonal) tTreg generation, meanwhile increasing this same self-antigen specific Tcon generation, despite an unchanged or increased total (polyclonal) tTreg population [105]. It will be interesting to see what further subtle implications the aging thymus has on central tolerance establishment via potentially altering certain self-tissue specific tTreg populations and altering the overall aged Treg TCR repertoire, in spite of a relatively increased aged polyclonal Treg population [92].

4.4 Overall contribution to inflammaging

Inflammaging or the age-related, persistent increase in basal pro-inflammatory phenotype, has long been thought to be primarily a result of senescent somatic cells exhibiting senescence-associated secretory phenotype (SASP) [30, 31, 34, 106]. However, it is has come to be appreciated that chronic immune activation in the elderly contributes to a pro-inflammatory secretory milieu. This activation in the elderly includes chronic innate immune activation, which may result from immunosenescence related to accumulation of memory T cells. Chronic innate immune activation is also attributed to long-term virus, such as cytomegalovirus (CMV) [29, 107, 108], infection; or a degeneration-associated autotoxic reaction [109]. However, age-related autoimmune predisposition (an adaptive immune activation), induced by adaptive immune reaction to self-tissues by self-reactive T cells, has recently been recognized as a potential factor and/or synergistic cause of chronic inflammation in the elderly [25, 34]. Therefore, the role of the adaptive immune system in mediating inflammaging, as a result of self-reactive T cell immune responses to self-tissue that increases with age, is directly related to the atrophied thymus [25, 34].

Since it has recently been confirmed that the involuted thymus releases self-reactive Tcon cells as a result of perturbed negative selection, the direct implications of age-related thymic atrophy on the risks of inflammaging and the associated subclinical increase in the pro-inflammatory milieu has become more clear [25].

Subsequent alterations in tTreg development may also play an unappreciated role in the increased self-reactivity associated with aging, as changes in the tTreg repertoire may in fact impair sufficient suppression of appropriate self-reactivity in the periphery, however, this still remains largely uninvestigated.

5. Trends in rejuvenation of age-related thymic atrophy

Rejuvenation of aged thymic function is one of the strategies to reduce inflammaging because it can reduce self-reactive Tcon cell release and potentially readjust tTreg cell function so that the adaptive immune aspects of inflammaging may be ameliorated. Several strategies to rejuvenate the atrophied thymus have been reported, including: (1) TEC stem cell-based strategies, including utilization of human embryonic/pluripotent stem cells [110–112], FoxN1$^{eGFP/+}$ knock-in epithelial cells [113], young TEC-based [114] or inducible TEC-based [115] strategies; (2) cytokine-to-TEC based therapy, such as keratinocyte growth factor (KGF) [116, 117] and IL-22 [118–120]; (3) genetically-based methods (enhancement of exogenous FoxN1 expression with FoxN1 cDNA plasmid and FoxN1 transgene) [79–81], and (4) epigenetically-based methods (via exosomes extracted from young healthy serum) [121].

As to the genetic rejuvenation strategy via exogenous FoxN1, intrathymic injection of plasmid vectors carrying FoxN1-cDNA into middle-aged and aged mice was able to partially rescue thymic atrophy and function. The investigators observed increased thymic size and thymocyte number in the treated group compared to mice receiving empty vector [79]. Another group utilized an inducible FoxN1 over-expression reporter gene system, and it was demonstrated that *in vivo* upregulation of FoxN1 expression in middle-aged and aged mice resulted in increased thymic size and thymocyte numbers as well as increased numbers of early thymic progenitor cells [81]. Additionally, the ratio of mTECs to cTECs, which is normally declined, was restored to normal levels [81].

As to cell-based therapy, this has also been investigated as a potential source of thymic rejuvenation via the use of exogenous TECs from newborn thymi. The investigators, after observing that circulating factors alone (via a heterochronic parabiosis model, in which young and aged mice are surgically joined resulting in mutual influence of blood-borne factors [122–130]) did not rejuvenate the aged thymus, utilized a model of direct transplantation of TECs from newborn mice intrathymically into middle-aged recipients [114]. This group observed renewed growth of the thymus as well as enhanced T cell generation [114].

Other groups are investigating the use of reprogrammed mouse embryonic fibroblasts (MEF), as sources of exogenous FoxN1, as a means of generating *de novo* ectopic thymus. One such group generated induced TECs (iTECs) from MEF cells by initiating FoxN1 expression that converted MEF cells into epithelial-like cells *in vitro* [115]. Then, these iTECs, after some testing, were re-aggregated and grafted under the kidney capsule of syngenic adult mice to evaluate the ability of these iTECs to develop into a functional thymus-like organ. Interestingly, the grafts were seeded by host T cell progenitors and reflected thymocyte distributions associated with the normal thymus at endpoint (4 weeks after engraftment). Additionally, typical thymus microstructure was observed in these grafts [115].

The overarching conclusions taken from these cytokine, cellular, genetic, or epigenetically-based rejuvenation strategies are that FoxN1 expression is a key target for rejuvenating TECs, resulting in a more functional thymus able to produce normal T cells. However, we need to recognize that any rejuvenation therapy has its pitfalls. For example, intrathymic injection of newborn TECs can rejuvenate middle-aged thymus [114], but the source of newborn TECs is limited and may not be ideal as a translational therapy. Additionally, generation of an ectopic *de novo* thymus under the kidney capsule [115] can generate naïve T cells, but this does not remedy the increased self-reactive T cells released by the original atrophied thymus remaining in the host. Also, the use of cytokines may help revitalize the thymus, but as a systemic therapy could present various detrimental side-effects. Therefore, further studies to develop practical and effective therapies are necessary.

6. Conclusion

In conclusion, age-related thymic atrophy is a dynamic process beginning early in life that shapes T cell development and the establishment of central T cell tolerance. There is substantial clinical significance in further exploring the underlying mechanisms of its effects on the various subsets of T cells developed in the atrophied thymus, namely Treg and Tcon cells. Also, continued investigation into potential avenues of thymic rejuvenation are striving to reverse the adverse effects of age-related thymic atrophy on the aged T cell immune system, since increased self-reactive T cells are observed with age, contributing to inflammaging. Moreover, there are numerous areas still to explore in this field with far-reaching applications.

Acknowledgements

We would like to thank Dr. Rance Berg (Department of Microbiology, Immunology and Genetics, UNTHSC) for critical reading of this manuscript.

Conflict of interest

The authors have no conflict of interest.

Funding

Supported by NIH/NIAID grant R01AI121147 to D-M. S. The funder had no role in study design, data collection and analysis, decision to publish, or preparation of the manuscript.

Author details

Rachel Thomas[1] and Dong-Ming Su[2]*

1 Cell Biology, Immunology, and Microbiology Graduate Program, Graduate School of Biomedical Sciences, University of North Texas Health Science Center, Fort Worth, Texas, USA

2 Department of Microbiology, Immunology, and Genetics, University of North Texas Health Science Center, Fort Worth, Texas, USA

*Address all correspondence to: dongming.su@unthsc.edu

References

[1] Kurd N, Robey EA. T-cell selection in the thymus: A spatial and temporal perspective. Immunological Reviews. 2016;**271**(1):114-126

[2] Palmer E. Negative selection—Clearing out the bad apples from the T-cell repertoire. Nature Reviews Immunology. 2003;**3**(5):383-391

[3] Hsieh CS, Lee HM, Lio CW. Selection of regulatory T cells in the thymus. Nature Reviews Immunology. 2012;**12**(3):157-167

[4] Cebula A, Seweryn M, Rempala GA, Pabla SS, McIndoe RA, Denning TL, et al. Thymus-derived regulatory T cells contribute to tolerance to commensal microbiota. Nature. 2013;**497**(7448):258-262

[5] Gallegos AM, Bevan MJ. Central tolerance: Good but imperfect. Immunological Reviews. 2006;**209**:290-296

[6] Rezzani R, Nardo L, Favero G, Peroni M, Rodella LF. Thymus and aging: Morphological, radiological, and functional overview. Age (Dordrecht, Netherlands). 2014;**36**(1):313-351

[7] Palmer DB. The effect of age on thymic function. Frontiers in Immunology. 2013;**4**:316

[8] Hale JS, Boursalian TE, Turk GL, Fink PJ. Thymic output in aged mice. Proceedings of the National Academy of Sciences of the United States of America. 2006;**103**(22):8447-8452

[9] Sudo K, Ema H, Morita Y, Nakauchi H. Age-associated characteristics of murine hematopoietic stem cells. The Journal of Experimental Medicine. 2000;**192**(9):1273-1280

[10] Min H, Montecino-Rodriguez E, Dorshkind K. Reduction in the developmental potential of intrathymic T cell progenitors with age. Journal of Immunology (Baltimore, Md. : 1950). 2004;**173**(1):245-250

[11] Kovtonyuk LV, Fritsch K, Feng X, Manz MG, Takizawa H. Inflamm-aging of Hematopoiesis, hematopoietic stem cells, and the bone marrow microenvironment. Frontiers in Immunology. 2016;**7**:502

[12] Latchney SE, Calvi LM. The aging hematopoietic stem cell niche: Phenotypic and functional changes and mechanisms that contribute to hematopoietic aging. Seminars in Hematology. 2017;**54**(1):25-32

[13] Sun L, Brown R, Chen S, Zhuge Q, Su DM. Aging induced decline in T-lymphopoiesis is primarily dependent on status of progenitor niches in the bone marrow and thymus. Aging. 2012;**4**(9):606-619

[14] Su DM, Aw D, Palmer DB. Immunosenescence: A product of the environment? Current Opinion in Immunology. 2013;**25**(4):498-503

[15] Anderson G, Jenkinson EJ. Lymphostromal interactions in thymic development and function. Nature Reviews. Immunology. 2001;**1**(1):31-40

[16] Vaidya HJ, Briones Leon A, Blackburn CC. FOXN1 in thymus organogenesis and development. European Journal of Immunology. 2016;**46**(8):1826-1837

[17] Pawelec G. Age and immunity: What is "immunosenescence"? Experimental Gerontology. 2018;**105**:4-9

[18] McElhaney JE, Effros RB. Immunosenescence: What does it mean to health outcomes in older adults?

Current Opinion in Immunology. 2009;**21**(4):418-424

[19] Pawelec G. Immunosenescence comes of age. Symposium on aging research in immunology: The impact of genomics. EMBO Reports. 2007;**8**(3):220-223

[20] Pawelec G, Wagner W, Adibzadeh M, Engel A. T cell immunosenescence in vitro and in vivo. Experimental Gerontology. 1999;**34**(3):419-429

[21] Nikolich-Zugich J. The twilight of immunity: Emerging concepts in aging of the immune system. Nature Immunology. 2018;**19**(1):10-19

[22] Zinger A, Cho WC, Ben-Yehuda A. Cancer and aging-the inflammatory connection. Aging and Disease. 2017;**8**(5):611-627

[23] Machiela MJ. Mosaicism, aging and cancer. Current Opinion in Oncology. 2019;**31**(2):108-113

[24] Xia J, Wang H, Guo J, Zhang Z, Coder B, Su DM. Age-related disruption of steady-state thymic medulla provokes autoimmune phenotype via perturbing negative selection. Aging and Disease. 2012;**3**(3):248-259

[25] Coder BD, Wang H, Ruan L, Su DM. Thymic involution perturbs negative selection leading to autoreactive T cells that induce chronic inflammation. Journal of Immunology (Baltimore, MD: 1950). 2015;**194**(12):5825-5837

[26] Coder B, Su DM. Thymic involution beyond T-cell insufficiency. Oncotarget. 2015;**6**(26):21777-21778

[27] De Martinis M, Franceschi C, Monti D, Ginaldi L. Inflammageing and lifelong antigenic load as major determinants of ageing rate and longevity. FEBS Letters. 2005;**579**(10):2035-2039

[28] Franceschi C, Bonafe M, Valensin S, Olivieri F, De Luca M, Ottaviani E, et al. Inflammaging. An evolutionary perspective on immunosenescence. Annals of the New York Academy of Sciences. 2000;**908**:244-254

[29] Brunner S, Herndler-Brandstetter D, Weinberger B, Grubeck-Loebenstein B. Persistent viral infections and immune aging. Ageing Research Reviews. 2011;**10**(3):362-369

[30] Freund A, Orjalo AV, Desprez PY, Campisi J. Inflammatory networks during cellular senescence: Causes and consequences. Trends in Molecular Medicine. 2010;**16**(5):238-246

[31] Franceschi C, Capri M, Monti D, Giunta S, Olivieri F, Sevini F, et al. Inflammaging and anti-inflammaging: A systemic perspective on aging and longevity emerged from studies in humans. Mechanisms of Ageing and Development. 2007;**128**(1):92-105

[32] Fulop T, Larbi A, Dupuis G, Le Page A, Frost EH, Cohen AA, et al. Immunosenescence and Inflamm-aging As two sides of the same coin: Friends or foes? Frontiers in Immunology. 2017;**8**:1960

[33] Gui J, Mustachio LM, Su DM, Craig RW. Thymus size and age-related thymic involution: Early programming, sexual dimorphism, progenitors and stroma. Aging and Disease. 2012;**3**(3):280-290

[34] Fulop T, Witkowski JM, Olivieri F, Larbi A. The integration of inflammaging in age-related diseases. Seminars in Immunology. 2018;**40**:17-35

[35] Palmer S, Albergante L, Blackburn CC, Newman TJ. Thymic involution and rising disease incidence with age. Proceedings of the National Academy of Sciences of the United States of America. 2018;**115**(8):1883-1888

[36] Aspinall R, Andrew D. Thymic involution in aging. Journal of Clinical Immunology. 2000;**20**(4):250-256

[37] Hinterberger M, Aichinger M, Prazeres da Costa O, Voehringer D, Hoffmann R, Klein L. Autonomous role of medullary thymic epithelial cells in central CD4(+) T cell tolerance. Nature Immunology. 2010;**11**(6):512-519

[38] Klein L, Kyewski B, Allen PM, Hogquist KA. Positive and negative selection of the T cell repertoire: What thymocytes see (and don't see). Nature Reviews Immunology. 2014;**14**(6):377-391

[39] Aw D, Silva AB, Maddick M, von Zglinicki T, Palmer DB. Architectural changes in the thymus of aging mice. Aging Cell. 2008;7(2):158-167

[40] Chinn IK, Blackburn CC, Manley NR, Sempowski GD. Changes in primary lymphoid organs with aging. Seminars in Immunology. 2012;**24**(5):309-320

[41] Burnley P, Rahman M, Wang H, Zhang Z, Sun X, Zhuge Q, et al. Role of the p63-FoxN1 regulatory axis in thymic epithelial cell homeostasis during aging. Cell Death & Disease. 2013;**4**:e932

[42] Masters AR, Haynes L, Su DM, Palmer DB. Immune senescence: Significance of the stromal microenvironment. Clinical and Experimental Immunology. 2017;**187**(1):6-15

[43] Sempowski GD, Hale LP, Sundy JS, Massey JM, Koup RA, Douek DC, et al. Leukemia inhibitory factor, oncostatin M, IL-6, and stem cell factor mRNA expression in human thymus increases with age and is associated with thymic atrophy. Journal of Immunology. 2000;**164**(4):2180-2187

[44] Pang WW, Price EA, Sahoo D, Beerman I, Maloney WJ, Rossi DJ, et al. Human bone marrow hematopoietic stem cells are increased in frequency and myeloid-biased with age. Proceedings of the National Academy of Sciences of the United States of America. 2011;**108**(50):20012-20017

[45] Linton PJ, Dorshkind K. Age-related changes in lymphocyte development and function. Nature Immunology. 2004;**5**(2):133-139

[46] Tyan ML. Age-related decrease in mouse T cell progenitors. Journal of Immunology (Baltimore, MD: 1950). 1977;**118**(3):846-851

[47] Morrison SJ, Wandycz AM, Akashi K, Globerson A, Weissman IL. The aging of hematopoietic stem cells. Nature Medicine. 1996;**2**(9):1011-1016

[48] Waterstrat A, Van Zant G. Effects of aging on hematopoietic stem and progenitor cells. Current Opinion in Immunology. 2009;**21**(4):408-413

[49] Van Zant G, Liang Y. Concise review: Hematopoietic stem cell aging, life span, and transplantation. Stem Cells Translational Medicine. 2012;**1**(9):651-657

[50] Min H, Montecino-Rodriguez E, Dorshkind K. Effects of aging on early B- and T-cell development. Immunological Reviews. 2005;**205**:7-17

[51] Zhu X, Gui J, Dohkan J, Cheng L, Barnes PF, Su DM. Lymphohematopoietic progenitors do not have a synchronized defect with age-related thymic involution. Aging Cell. 2007;**6**(5):663-672

[52] Peschon JJ, Morrissey PJ, Grabstein KH, Ramsdell FJ, Maraskovsky E, Gliniak BC, et al. Early lymphocyte expansion is severely impaired in interleukin 7 receptor-deficient mice. The Journal of Experimental Medicine. 1994;**180**(5):1955-1960

[53] Sun L, Hurez VJ, Thibodeaux SR, Kious MJ, Liu A, Lin P, et al. Aged regulatory T cells protect from autoimmune inflammation despite reduced STAT3 activation and decreased constraint of IL-17 producing T cells. Aging Cell. 2012;**11**(3):509-519

[54] Porritt HE, Rumfelt LL, Tabrizifard S, Schmitt TM, Zuniga-Pflucker JC, Petrie HT. Heterogeneity among DN1 prothymocytes reveals multiple progenitors with different capacities to generate T cell and non-T cell lineages. Immunity. 2004;**20**(6):735-745

[55] Gui J, Zhu X, Dohkan J, Cheng L, Barnes PF, Su DM. The aged thymus shows normal recruitment of lymphohematopoietic progenitors but has defects in thymic epithelial cells. International Immunology. 2007;**19**(10):1201-1211

[56] Aspinall R, Andrew D. Thymic atrophy in the mouse is a soluble problem of the thymic environment. Vaccine. 2000;**18**(16):1629-1637

[57] Henson SM, Snelgrove R, Hussell T, Wells DJ, Aspinall R. An IL-7 fusion protein that shows increased thymopoietic ability. Journal of Immunology (Baltimore, MD: 1950). 2005;**175**(6):4112-4118

[58] van Ewijk W, Hollander G, Terhorst C, Wang B. Stepwise development of thymic microenvironments in vivo is regulated by thymocyte subsets. Development. 2000;**127**(8):1583-1591

[59] Shores EW, Van Ewijk W, Singer A. Disorganization and restoration of thymic medullary epithelial cells in T cell receptor-negative scid mice: Evidence that receptor-bearing lymphocytes influence maturation of the thymic microenvironment. European Journal of Immunology. 1991;**21**(7):1657-1661

[60] Stanger BZ, Tanaka AJ, Melton DA. Organ size is limited by the number of embryonic progenitor cells in the pancreas but not the liver. Nature. 2007;**445**(7130):886-891

[61] Jenkinson WE, Bacon A, White AJ, Anderson G, Jenkinson EJ. An epithelial progenitor pool regulates thymus growth. Journal of Immunology. 2008;**181**(9):6101-6108

[62] Foss DL, Donskoy E, Goldschneider I. The importation of hematogenous precursors by the thymus is a gated phenomenon in normal adult mice. The Journal of Experimental Medicine. 2001;**193**(3):365-374

[63] Donskoy E, Foss D, Goldschneider I. Gated importation of prothymocytes by adult mouse thymus is coordinated with their periodic mobilization from bone marrow. Journal of Immunology. 2003;**171**(7):3568-3575

[64] Moore KA, Lemischka IR. Stem cells and their niches. Science. 2006;**311**(5769):1880-1885

[65] Wilson A, Trumpp A. Bone-marrow haematopoietic-stem-cell niches. Nature Reviews. Immunology. 2006;**6**(2):93-106

[66] Prockop SE, Petrie HT. Regulation of thymus size by competition for stromal niches among early T cell progenitors. Journal of Immunology. 2004;**173**(3):1604-1611

[67] Nehls M, Pfeifer D, Schorpp M, Hedrich H, Boehm T. New member of the winged-helix protein family disrupted in mouse and rat nude mutations. Nature. 1994;**372**(6501):103-107

[68] Nehls M, Kyewski B, Messerle M, Waldschutz R, Schuddekopf K, Smith AJ, et al. Two genetically separable steps in the differentiation

of thymic epithelium. Science. 1996;**272**(5263):886-889

[69] Schlake T. The nude gene and the skin. Experimental Dermatology. 2001;**10**(5):293-304

[70] Brissette JL, Li J, Kamimura J, Lee D, Dotto GP. The product of the mouse nude locus, Whn, regulates the balance between epithelial cell growth and differentiation. Genes & Development. 1996;**10**(17):2212-2221

[71] Flanagan SP. 'Nude', a new hairless gene with pleiotropic effects in the mouse. Genetical Research. 1966;**8**(3):295-309

[72] Pantelouris EM. Absence of thymus in a mouse mutant. Nature. 1968;**217**(5126):370-371

[73] Ortman CL, Dittmar KA, Witte PL, Le PT. Molecular characterization of the mouse involuted thymus: Aberrations in expression of transcription regulators in thymocyte and epithelial compartments. International Immunology. 2002;**14**(7):813-822

[74] Rode I, Martins VC, Kublbeck G, Maltry N, Tessmer C, Rodewald HR. FoxN1 protein expression in the developing, aging, and regenerating Thymus. Journal of Immunology. 2015;**195**(12):5678-5687

[75] Cheng L, Guo J, Sun L, Fu J, Barnes PF, Metzger D, et al. Postnatal tissue-specific disruption of transcription factor FoxN1 triggers acute thymic atrophy. The Journal of Biological Chemistry. 2010;**285**(8):5836-5847

[76] Zhang Z, Burnley P, Coder B, Su DM. Insights on FoxN1 biological significance and usages of the "nude" mouse in studies of T-lymphopoiesis. International Journal of Biological Sciences. 2012;**8**(8):1156-1167

[77] Matsuda T, Cepko CL. Controlled expression of transgenes introduced by in vivo electroporation. Proceedings of the National Academy of Sciences of the United States of America. 2007;**104**(3):1027-1032

[78] Bleul CC, Corbeaux T, Reuter A, Fisch P, Monting JS, Boehm T. Formation of a functional thymus initiated by a postnatal epithelial progenitor cell. Nature. 2006;**441**(7096):992-996

[79] Sun L, Guo J, Brown R, Amagai T, Zhao Y, Su DM. Declining expression of a single epithelial cell-autonomous gene accelerates age-related thymic involution. Aging Cell. 2010;**9**(3):347-357

[80] Zook EC, Krishack PA, Zhang S, Zeleznik-Le NJ, Firulli AB, Witte PL, et al. Overexpression of FoxN1 attenuates age-associated thymic involution and prevents the expansion of peripheral CD4 memory T cells. Blood. 2011;**118**(22):5723-5731

[81] Bredenkamp N, Nowell CS, Blackburn CC. Regeneration of the aged thymus by a single transcription factor. Development (Cambridge, England). 2014;**141**(8):1627-1637

[82] O'Neill KE, Bredenkamp N, Tischner C, Vaidya HJ, Stenhouse FH, Peddie CD, et al. FoxN1 is dynamically regulated in thymic epithelial cells during embryogenesis and at the onset of thymic involution. PLoS One. 2016;**11**(3):e0151666

[83] Swain S, Clise-Dwyer K, Haynes L. Homeostasis and the age-associated defect of CD4 T cells. Seminars in Immunology. 2005;**17**(5):370-377

[84] Goronzy JJ, Lee WW, Weyand CM. Aging and T-cell diversity. Experimental Gerontology. 2007;**42**(5):400-406

[85] Petrie HT. Role of thymic organ structure and stromal composition in steady-state postnatal T-cell production. Immunological Reviews. 2002;**189**:8-19

[86] Hodes RJ. Telomere length, aging, and somatic cell turnover. The Journal of Experimental Medicine. 1999;**190**(2):153-156

[87] Franceschi C, Valensin S, Fagnoni F, Barbi C, Bonafe M. Biomarkers of immunosenescence within an evolutionary perspective: The challenge of heterogeneity and the role of antigenic load. Experimental Gerontology. 1999;**34**(8):911-921

[88] Guo J, Feng Y, Barnes P, Huang FF, Idell S, Su DM, et al. Deletion of FoxN1 in the thymic medullary epithelium reduces peripheral T cell responses to infection and mimics changes of aging. PLoS One. 2012;**7**(4):e34681

[89] Stritesky GL, Jameson SC, Hogquist KA. Selection of self-reactive T cells in the thymus. Annual Review of Immunology. 2012;**30**:95-114

[90] Josefowicz SZ, Lu LF, Rudensky AY. Regulatory T cells: Mechanisms of differentiation and function. Annual Review of Immunology. 2012;**30**:531-564

[91] Li MO, Rudensky AY. T cell receptor signalling in the control of regulatory T cell differentiation and function. Nature Reviews Immunology. 2016;**16**(4):220-233

[92] Oh J, Wang W, Thomas R, Su DM. Capacity of tTreg generation is not impaired in the atrophied thymus. PLoS Biology. 2017;**15**(11):e2003352

[93] Klein L, Robey EA, Hsieh CS. Central CD4(+) T cell tolerance: Deletion versus regulatory T cell differentiation. Nature Reviews. Immunology. 2019;**19**(1):7-18

[94] Pohar J, Simon Q, Fillatreau S. Antigen-specificity in the thymic development and peripheral activity of CD4(+)FOXP3(+) T regulatory cells. Frontiers in Immunology. 2018;**9**:1701

[95] Lathrop SK, Santacruz NA, Pham D, Luo J, Hsieh CS. Antigen-specific peripheral shaping of the natural regulatory T cell population. The Journal of Experimental Medicine. 2008;**205**(13):3105-3117

[96] Wirnsberger G, Hinterberger M, Klein L. Regulatory T-cell differentiation versus clonal deletion of autoreactive thymocytes. Immunology and Cell Biology. 2011;**89**(1):45-53

[97] Malek TR, Bayer AL. Tolerance, not immunity, crucially depends on IL-2. Nature Reviews Immunology. 2004;**4**(9):665-674

[98] Liu Y, Zhang P, Li J, Kulkarni AB, Perruche S, Chen W. A critical function for TGF-beta signaling in the development of natural CD4+CD25+Foxp3+ regulatory T cells. Nature Immunology. 2008;**9**(6):632-640

[99] Konkel JE, Jin W, Abbatiello B, Grainger JR, Chen W. Thymocyte apoptosis drives the intrathymic generation of regulatory T cells. Proceedings of the National Academy of Sciences of the United States of America. 2014;**111**(4):E465-E473

[100] Hwang S, Song KD, Lesourne R, Lee J, Pinkhasov J, Li L, et al. Reduced TCR signaling potential impairs negative selection but does not result in autoimmune disease. The Journal of Experimental Medicine. 2012;**209**(10):1781-1795

[101] Leonard JD, Gilmore DC, Dileepan T, Nawrocka WI, Chao JL, Schoenbach MH, et al. Identification of natural regulatory T cell epitopes reveals convergence on a dominant autoantigen. Immunity. 2017;**47**(1):107.e8-117.e8

[102] Malchow S, Leventhal DS, Savage PA. Organ-specific regulatory T cells of thymic origin are expanded in murine prostate tumors. Oncoimmunology. 2013;**2**(7):e24898

[103] Malchow S, Leventhal DS, Lee V, Nishi S, Socci ND, Savage PA. Aire enforces immune tolerance by directing autoreactive T cells into the regulatory T cell lineage. Immunity. 2016;**44**(5):1102-1113

[104] Kieback E, Hilgenberg E, Stervbo U, Lampropoulou V, Shen P, Bunse M, et al. Thymus-derived regulatory T cells are positively selected on natural self-antigen through cognate interactions of High functional avidity. Immunity. 2016;**44**(5):1114-1126

[105] Lages CS, Suffia I, Velilla PA, Huang B, Warshaw G, Hildeman DA, et al. Functional regulatory T cells accumulate in aged hosts and promote chronic infectious disease reactivation. Journal of Immunology (Baltimore, MD: 1950). 2008;**181**(3):1835-1848

[106] Campisi J. Cellular senescence: Putting the paradoxes in perspective. Current Opinion in Genetics & Development. 2011;**21**(1):107-112

[107] Nikolich-Zugich J. Ageing and life-long maintenance of T-cell subsets in the face of latent persistent infections. Nature Reviews. Immunology. 2008;**8**(7):512-522

[108] High KP, Akbar AN, Nikolich-Zugich J. Translational research in immune senescence: Assessing the relevance of current models. Seminars in Immunology. 2012;**24**(5):373-382

[109] McGeer PL, McGeer EG. Inflammation and the degenerative diseases of aging. Annals of the New York Academy of Sciences. 2004;**1035**:104-116

[110] Parent AV, Russ HA, Khan IS, LaFlam TN, Metzger TC, Anderson MS, et al. Generation of functional thymic epithelium from human embryonic stem cells that supports host T cell development. Cell Stem Cell. 2013;**13**(2): 219-229

[111] Sun X, Xu J, Lu H, Liu W, Miao Z, Sui X, et al. Directed differentiation of human embryonic stem cells into thymic epithelial progenitor-like cells reconstitutes the thymic microenvironment in vivo. Cell Stem Cell. 2013;**13**(2):230-236

[112] Soh CL, Giudice A, Jenny RA, Elliott DA, Hatzistavrou T, Micallef SJ, et al. FoxN1 (GFP/w) reporter hESCs enable identification of integrin-beta4, HLA-DR, and EpCAM as markers of human PSC-derived FoxN1(+) thymic epithelial progenitors. Stem Cell Reports. 2014;**2**(6):925-937

[113] Barsanti M, Lim JM, Hun ML, Lister N, Wong K, Hammett MV, et al. A novel FoxN1(eGFP/+) mouse model identifies Bmp4-induced maintenance of FoxN1 expression and thymic epithelial progenitor populations. European Journal of Immunology. 2017;**47**(2):291-304

[114] Kim MJ, Miller CM, Shadrach JL, Wagers AJ, Serwold T. Young, proliferative thymic epithelial cells engraft and function in aging thymuses. Journal of Immunology (Baltimore, MD: 1950). 2015;**194**(10):4784-4795

[115] Bredenkamp N, Ulyanchenko S, O'Neill KE, Manley NR, Vaidya HJ, Blackburn CC. An organized and functional thymus generated from FoxN1-reprogrammed fibroblasts. Nature Cell Biology. 2014;**16**(9):902-908

[116] Erickson M, Morkowski S, Lehar S, Gillard G, Beers C, Dooley J, et al. Regulation of thymic epithelium by keratinocyte growth factor. Blood. 2002;**100**(9):3269-3278

[117] Alpdogan O, Hubbard VM, Smith OM, Patel N, Lu S, Goldberg GL, et al. Keratinocyte growth factor (KGF) is required for postnatal thymic regeneration. Blood. 2006;**107**(6):2453-2460

[118] Bhandoola A, Artis D. Immunology. Rebuilding the thymus. Science. 2012;**336**(6077):40-41

[119] Dudakov JA, Hanash AM, Jenq RR, Young LF, Ghosh A, Singer NV, et al. Interleukin-22 drives endogenous thymic regeneration in mice. Science. 2012;**336**(6077):91-95

[120] Chaudhry MS, Velardi E, Dudakov JA, van den Brink MR. Thymus: The next (re)generation. Immunological Reviews. 2016;**271**(1):56-71

[121] Wang W, Wang L, Ruan L, Oh J, Dong X, Zhuge Q, et al. Extracellular vesicles extracted from young donor serum attenuate inflammaging via partially rejuvenating aged T-cell immunotolerance. FASEB Journal: Official Publication of the Federation of American Societies for Experimental Biology. 2018;**32**(11):5899-5912. DOI: 10.1096/fj201800059R

[122] Conboy IM, Conboy MJ, Wagers AJ, Girma ER, Weissman IL, Rando TA. Rejuvenation of aged progenitor cells by exposure to a young systemic environment. Nature. 2005;**433**(7027):760-764

[123] Pishel I, Shytikov D, Orlova T, Peregudov A, Artyuhov I, Butenko G. Accelerated aging versus rejuvenation of the immune system in heterochronic parabiosis. Rejuvenation Research. 2012;**15**(2):239-248

[124] Ruckh JM, Zhao JW, Shadrach JL, van Wijngaarden P, Rao TN, Wagers AJ, et al. Rejuvenation of regeneration in the aging central nervous system. Cell Stem Cell. 2012;**10**(1):96-103

[125] Brack AS, Conboy MJ, Roy S, Lee M, Kuo CJ, Keller C, et al. Increased Wnt signaling during aging alters muscle stem cell fate and increases fibrosis. Science. 2007;**317**(5839):807-810

[126] Loffredo FS, Steinhauser ML, Jay SM, Gannon J, Pancoast JR, Yalamanchi P, et al. Growth differentiation factor 11 is a circulating factor that reverses age-related cardiac hypertrophy. Cell. 2013;**153**(4):828-839

[127] Katsimpardi L, Litterman NK, Schein PA, Miller CM, Loffredo FS, Wojtkiewicz GR, et al. Vascular and neurogenic rejuvenation of the aging mouse brain by young systemic factors. Science. 2014;**344**(6184):630-634

[128] Villeda SA, Plambeck KE, Middeldorp J, Castellano JM, Mosher KI, Luo J, et al. Young blood reverses age-related impairments in cognitive function and synaptic plasticity in mice. Nature Medicine. Jun 2014;**20**(6):659-663

[129] Villeda SA, Luo J, Mosher KI, Zou B, Britschgi M, Bieri G, et al. The ageing systemic milieu negatively regulates neurogenesis and cognitive function. Nature. 2011;**477**(7362):90-94

[130] Villeda SA, Wyss-Coray T. The circulatory systemic environment as a modulator of neurogenesis and brain aging. Autoimmunity Reviews. 2013;**12**(6):674-677

Chapter 6

Congenital Anomalies of the Thymus

Ali Kouhi and Saeed Sohrabpour

Abstract

The thymus, a retrosternal lymphoid tissue, develops from the third and fourth pharyngeal pouches like the parathyroid glands at the sixth week of gestational age. The thymus is usually located in the anterior mediastinum, although it can be found anywhere in the thymopharyngeal path. The thymus has a bilobed or quadrilateral shape; however, it can be found in other shapes. Limited information is available about the precise epidemiology of thymic congenital anomalies. Since these anomalies are not symptomatic, it may be more common than the available reports. There are various reports available about the prevalence of thymic diseases and anomalies ranging from 4.45 to 30%. In this chapter we tried to have a review on epidemiology, definition, and management of congenital anomalies of the thymus.

Keywords: thymic gland, congenital anomalies, epidemiology, treatments

1. History

The word "thymus" is originally derived from the Greek word "thumos" which means "soul." Previously, in the ancient world, it was believed that the soul is located in this organ. The function of the thymus was a mystery for centuries. The first who defined a role for the thymus was Galen in the second century AD. He believed that the thymus has the responsibility for purification of the nervous system [1, 2]. Later in the fifteenth century, Vesalius mentioned that the thymus works as a shield for protection of major vessels located behind the sternum [2]. The thymus was known as the regulator of fetal and neonatal pulmonary function [1, 2]. For the first time, the thymus was identified as a lymph modifying gland in 1777 by William Hewson. Dissection of corpses let Sir Astley Cooper to write an entire book about the anatomy of the thymus gland [3]. Hassall and Vanarsdale made a remarkable progress in our knowledge about the thymus in 1846 describing the differences between other lymphoid organs and the thymus [4]. Back at the beginning of the twentieth century, finding a relatively large mass (thymus) in autopsy of children who died because of diphtheria was not a fortune. Physicians believed that a smaller thymus presents a normal one [5]. So, some of them used to prescribe radiation therapy for reducing the size of the thymus which resulted in thyroid adenocarcinoma in most of the cases [6]. In 1961, Miller showed the true function of the thymus by describing its destructing effect on the immune system [2, 3].

2. Development of the thymus

The thymus, a retrosternal lymphoid tissue, develops from the third and fourth pharyngeal pouches like the parathyroid glands at the sixth week of gestational age [7–10]. During the next weeks of development, the thymus migrates through a path, called thymopharyngeal duct, to its final destiny which is the anterior mediastinum [11]. The liver and bone marrow are the primary organs responsible for production of lymphoid cells. These cells migrate to the thymus gland which results in differentiation of the thymus into a cortex and medulla [7].

The thymus is usually located in the anterior mediastinum, although it can be found anywhere in the thymopharyngeal path. The thymus has a bilobed or quadrilateral shape; however, it can be found in other shapes. The thymus is commonly found in chest radiographs of infants and children as a large mediastinal mass. During adolescence, the thymus encounters a fibrofatty change as the age increases. Growth of the thymus continues from birth to 2–3 years of age, when it reaches its highest weight, while sex hormones make the thymus smaller during adolescence. Appropriate function of the thymus in childhood guarantees the condition of the immune system [12].

3. Epidemiology of congenital anomalies of the thymus

Limited information is available about the precise epidemiology of thymic congenital anomalies. Since these anomalies are not symptomatic, it may be more common than the available reports [13–15]. There are various reports available about the prevalence of thymic diseases and anomalies ranging from 4.45 to 30% [16–18]. It could be concluded that thymic anomalies are common, but their symptomatic manifestation is uncommon. According to the previous studies, thymic congenital anomalies and diseases are three times more prevalent in men than women [13]. Also it has been reported that two thirds of these lesions are usually found in the first decade of life [19]; the oldest reported age of presentation is 71.

3.1 Thymic cyst

As one of the uncommon lesions of the thymus gland, thymic cysts may be seen in various age groups. Congenital forms of thymic cysts can be found anywhere along with the thymopharyngeal path. In addition, thymic cysts may be developed following thoracotomy or chemotherapy [20]. In imaging, these lesions have a thin wall with no solid components and do not enhance with intravenous contrast administration. These cysts may contain protein or hemorrhagic fluid. On histologic examination, the wall of cyst is lined by the columnar or stratified epithelium.

3.2 Ectopic cervical thymus

The exact incidence of ectopic cervical thymus remains unclear because of the asymptomatic nature of these masses. Cervical thymus is usually detected incidentally [21, 22]. Ultrasonography is the choice method for imaging especially in children requiring no contrast or sedation. Echo characteristics of an aberrant cervical thymus are easily defined by ultrasonography. Ultrasonic features of cervical thymus, echogenic linear structures surrounded by hypoechoic rims, are similar to those of the mediastinal thymus [23, 24]. In cases with large ectopic thymus, diagnosis is more challenging where fine needle aspiration cytology may be helpful.

3.3 Undescended thymus

As a rare lesion, undescended thymus is usually presented as a midline neck swelling in a child. Thyroglossal duct cyst, thyroid or parathyroid lesions, and cystic hygroma or cystic teratoma are among other differential diagnoses. A variety of imaging modalities are useful for diagnosing undescended thymus such as MRI, nuclear scan (Gallium 61), computed tomography, ultrasonography, or conventional radiography [25].

3.4 Thymopharyngeal duct cyst

Thymopharyngeal duct cyst, also known as thymic remnant cyst (TRC), is one of the rare lesions of the thymus gland [26]. A majority of these cysts occur in the first decade of life and on the left side of the neck [27]. These cysts may be completely separated from the normal thymic tissue or attached to the thymus [28]. CT scan shows TRCs as a cyst with thin wall. After administration of contrast, thymic remnant cysts show peripheral rim enhancement [29]. Malformations of the lymphatic system, external laryngocele, lymphadenopathy, vallecular cyst, cystic neuroblastoma, and thyroglossal cyst are among differential diagnoses of TRCs [30]. It is very important to differentiate TRCs with the second branchial cleft anomalies as they require different treatment approaches.

4. Physiology of the thymus

The thymus plays the main role in the development of the immune system during infancy and childhood [15]. The thymus gland has the responsibility for implying differentiation of CD4 and CD8 T cells. It also proliferates clones of mature T cells for entering the lymph flow and developing immune tolerance resulting in prevention of autoimmune diseases. On the other hand, the thymus is involved in secretion of hormones such as thymulin, thymosin alpha 1, and thymopentin [2–4].

5. Treatment

Surgery is the choice method for diagnosis and treatment of symptomatic thymic gland masses. Ectopic thymic lesions are usually treated by complete surgical resection even in the absence of evident malignancy. Some malignant transformations have been reported in cases with solid ectopic thymic tissue and thymoma in cervical ectopic thymus [31–33].

With the important role of the thymus gland in the immune system, surgeons should make sure about the presence of a mediastinal thymus before thymectomy [34]. Some authors have mentioned that benign thymic lesions can be treated by conservative management; however, a surgical procedure should be considered if further changes are noticed in further studies [29]. Thymic cysts should be completely resected as they contain no active thymic tissue.

Author details

Ali Kouhi[1*] and Saeed Sohrabpour[2]

1 Otorhinolaryngology Research Center, Department of Otolaryngology-Head and Neck Surgery, Tehran University of Medical Sciences, Tehran, Iran

2 Otorhinolaryngology Research Center, Tehran University of Medical Sciences, Tehran, Iran

*Address all correspondence to: ali.kouhi@gmail.com

References

[1] Jacobs MT, Frush DP, Donnelly LF. The right place at the wrong time: Historical perspective of the relation of the thymus gland and pediatric radiology. Radiology. 1999;**210**(1):11-16

[2] Miller JF. The discovery of thymus function and of thymus-derived lymphocytes. Immunological Reviews. 2002;**185**(1):7-14

[3] Ribatti D, Crivellato E, Vacca A. Miller's seminal studies on the role of thymus in immunity. Clinical & Experimental Immunology. 2006;**144**(3):371-375

[4] Kappler JW, Roehm N, Marrack P. T cell tolerance by clonal elimination in the thymus. Cell. 1987;**49**(2):273-280

[5] Haley PJ. Species differences in the structure and function of the immune system. Toxicology. 2003;**188**(1):49-71

[6] Wolstenholme GE, Knight J. The immunologically competent cell, its nature and origin. Academic Medicine. 1 Oct 1964;**39**(10):976

[7] Nishino M, Ashiku SK, Kocher ON, Thurer RL, Boiselle PM, Hatabu H. The thymus: A comprehensive review. Radiographics. 2006;**26**(2):335-348

[8] Nasseri F, Eftekhari F. Clinical and radiologic review of the normal and abnormal thymus: Pearls and pitfalls. Radiographics. 2010;**30**(2):413-428

[9] Ge Q, Zhao Y. Evolution of thymus organogenesis. Developmental & Comparative Immunology. 2013;**39**(1-2):85-90

[10] Lele SM, Lele MS, Anderson VM. The thymus in infancy and childhood. Embryologic, anatomic, and pathologic considerations. Chest Surgery Clinics of North America. 2001;**11**(2):233-253. ix

[11] Goldstein AJ, Oliva I, Honarpisheh H, Rubinowitz A. A tour of the thymus: A review of thymic lesions with radiologic and pathologic correlation. Canadian Association of Radiologists Journal. 2015;**66**(1):5-15

[12] Elmore SA. Enhanced histopathology of the thymus. Toxicologic Pathology. 2006;**34**(5):656-665

[13] Petropoulos I, Konstantinidis I, Noussios G, Karagiannidis K, Kontzoglou G. Thymic cyst in the differential diagnosis of paediatric cervical masses. B-ENT. 2006;**2**(1):35-37

[14] Liu D, Kitajima M, Awai K, Nakayama Y, Tamura Y, Suda H, et al. Ectopic cervical thymus in an infant. Radiation Medicine. 2006;**24**(6):452-455

[15] Prasad T, Chui C, Ong C, Meenakshi A. Cervical ectopic thymus in an infant. Singapore Medical Journal. 2006;**47**(1):68

[16] Wagner CW, Vinocur CD, Weintraub WH, Golladay ES. Respiratory complications in cervical thymic cysts. Journal of Pediatric Surgery. 1988;**23**(7):657-660

[17] Pages A, Girardot B. Cervical thymic choristoma. In: Annales de Pathologie. Vol. 13. 1993. pp. 164-169

[18] Tabatabaie SA, Hashemi SM, Sanei B, Sanei MH. The frequency of ectopic thymic tissue in the necks of patients without any thymic disease. Medical Science Monitor. 2007;**13**(6):CR283-CRCR5

[19] Khariwala S, Nicollas R, Triglia J, Garabedian E, Marianowski R, Van Den Abbeele T, et al. Cervical presentations of thymic anomalies in children. International Journal of Pediatric Otorhinolaryngology. 2004;**68**(7):909-914

[20] Vinay K, Abbas AK, Fauston N. Robbins and cotran pathologic basis of disease. China: Saunders, Elsevier; 2005;**8**:208-221

[21] Ünal E, Düzkalir HG, Kurt-Güney S, Isildak ET. Aberrant cervical thymus and the role of ultrasonography: A case report. The Turkish Journal of Pediatrics. 2016;**58**(2):230

[22] Zielke AM, Swischuk LE, Hernandez JA. Ectopic cervical thymic tissue: Can imaging obviate biopsy and surgical removal? Pediatric Radiology. 2007;**37**(11):1174-1177

[23] Han BK, Yoon H-K, Suh Y-L. Thymic ultrasound: II. Diagnosis of aberrant cervical thymus. Pediatric Radiology. 2001;**31**(7)

[24] Song I, Yoo S-Y, Kim J, Hong E, Yoon H-K. Aberrant cervical thymus: Imaging and clinical findings in 13 children. Clinical Radiology. 2011;**66**(1):38-42

[25] Sherwani P, Pahwa S, Singhal S, Narula MK. Undescended thymus: A rare cause of midline neck swelling. The Indian Journal of Pediatrics. 2014;**81**(12):1425-1426

[26] Cigliano B, Baltogiannis N, De Marco M, Faviou E, Antoniou D, De Luca U, et al. Cervical thymic cysts. Pediatric Surgery International. 2007;**23**(12):1219-1225

[27] Reiner M, Beck AR, Rybak B. Cervical thymic cysts in children. The American Journal of Surgery. 1980;**139**(5):704-707

[28] Nguyen Q, deTar M, Wells W, Crockett D. Cervical thymic cyst: Case reports and review of the literature. The Laryngoscope. 1996;**106**(3):247-252

[29] Kelley DJ, Gerber ME, Willging JP. Cervicomediastinal thymic cysts. International Journal of Pediatric Otorhinolaryngology. 1997;**39**(2):139-146

[30] JC E. Paediatric head and neck imaging. In: John R, Haaga LC, Gilkeson RC, editors. CT and MR Imaging of the Whole Body. Missouri: Mosby; 2003. pp. 695-696

[31] Hernández ÁAH, Valderrama PA, Pérez JAD. Congenital anomalies of thymic origin in the neck. Acta Otorrinolaringologica (English Edition). 2008;**59**(5):244-249

[32] Miyauchi A, Kuma K, Matsuzuka F, Matsubayashi S, Kobayashi A, Tamai H, et al. Intrathyroidal epithelial thymoma: An entity distinct from squamous cell carcinoma of the thyroid. World Journal of Surgery. 1985;**9**(1):128-134

[33] Kakudo K, Mori I, Tamaoki N, Watanabe K. Carcinoma of possible thymic origin presenting as a thyroid mass: A new subgroup of squamous cell carcinoma of the thyroid. Journal of Surgical Oncology. 1988;**38**(3):187-192

[34] Madhok AB, Chandrasekran A, Parnell V, Gandhi M, Chowdhury D, Pahwa S. Levels of recent thymic emigrant cells decrease in children undergoing partial thymectomy during cardiac surgery. Clinical and Diagnostic Laboratory Immunology. 2005;**12**(5):563-565

Chapter 7

Thymoma and Thymic Carcinoma

Annette Rebecca Bijsmans and Robin Cornelissen

Abstract

Malignancies of the thymus are a rare entity and are often without local symptoms. However, paraneoplastic syndromes can give symptoms varying from very mild to life-threatening. The diagnostic workup and management of these tumors warrant a multidisciplinary approach. Treatment choice is mainly decided upon by pathological World Health Organization (WHO) subtype and clinical staging. In contrast to historical belief, biopsy could be considered when indicated. For resectable tumors, surgical approach is advised, with adjuvant radiotherapy for Masaoka-Koga stage III tumors. Whether Masaoka-Koga stage II tumors should be treated with radiotherapy is controversial given different outcomes in multiple studies. In Masaoka-Koga stage III, combinations with induction chemotherapy are the standard. A surgical approach should be considered even in stage IVa disease. If distant metastases are present, the patient can be treated with systemic chemotherapy. Despite many phase II studies having been published, there is no randomized controlled phase III data regarding optimal treatment available. In addition to chemotherapy, sunitinib and octreotide have been described to be effective. Immunotherapy is seen as Pandora's box given the possibility of immune-related side effects in this immunological organ. All known data regarding immunotherapy will be discussed.

Keywords: thymoma, thymic carcinoma, autoimmune paraneoplastic syndromes, surgery, radiation, chemotherapy, immunotherapy, targeted therapy

1. Introduction

Malignancies of the thymus are rare accounting for <1% of all adult neoplasms. Thymoma and thymus carcinoma account for 20% of tumors in the anterior mediastinum and are therefore the most commonly found malignancy in that specific location.

There are several groups of thymic tumors to distinguish thymic epithelial tumors, germ cell tumors, lymphoid and hematological malignancies, and mesenchymal tumors. It is known that they derive from or differentiate toward thymic cellular components, but the etiology of thymic neoplasms is largely unknown [1].

This chapter is about the epithelial tumors thymoma and thymic carcinoma (which include the neuroendocrine tumors). These tumors are histologically characterized by thymic stroma and lymphocytes. Thymomas usually exhibit a slow growth pattern, but they do have malignant potential and show a propensity for local invasion and intrathoracic recurrence. Extrathoracic metastases of thymomas are quite rare [2]. Thymic carcinomas are more aggressive, with invasion in the surrounding mediastinal structures. Extrathoracic metastases occur in <7% of patients [3]. Although thymomas and thymic carcinomas arise mostly in the anterior mediastinum, they can also be found in other mediastinal compartments, as well as in the neck, lung, pleura, and thyroid, due to ectopic thymic tissue [1, 4, 5].

Approximately 1000 new cases are diagnosed per year in Europe [6]. Patients are usually between 20 and 70 years of age, with a peak in 30–40 years for those with myasthenia gravis and 60–70 years for those without myasthenia gravis. Incidence is similar in men and women [3, 7]. There are no known risk factors [3, 7], although clusters of thymoma are described in patients with multiple endocrine neoplasia type 1 (MEN1) syndrome [8] and an association between the Epstein–Barr virus and myasthenia gravis in thymoma patients has been suggested [9].

2. WHO histological classification

Numerous classifications for thymic neoplasms, based on different histological and clinical criteria, have been proposed in the past. For universal agreement purposes, the International Committee of the World Health Organization (WHO) developed a classification system that distinguishes five histological subtypes of thymomas that differ in both morphological and clinical presentation and which correlate with invasion [1]. The WHO classification is increasingly more malignant from A to B3. Thymomas are composed of a mixture of neoplastic epithelial cells and normal T lymphocytes and exhibit a resemblance to the normal thymic architecture, which cannot be found in other organs. In contrast, thymic carcinoma (in the past considered as a thymoma type C) is similar to carcinomas found outside the thymus. Although most thymomas have an excellent prognosis, they can be locally invasive and are (although rarely) able to spread to lymph nodes or extrathoracic sites, so the term "benign" should be avoided.

Type A thymoma is composed of spindle cells and a few to no lymphocytes. About 24% of the type A thymomas are found in patients suffering from myasthenia gravis, and pure red cell aplasia may occur. Eighty percent of type A thymomas are Masaoka-Koga stage I on presentation (for explanation on the Masaoka-Koga staging system, see paragraph on staging). Stage IV is rare in this histological subtype [1, 3]. The prognosis of type A thymoma is excellent with 5- and 10-year survival rates close to 100% [10].

Type AB thymoma is composed of a mixture of lymphocyte-poor type A thymoma and more lymphocyte-rich type B. Approximately 14% of type AB thymomas are associated with the development of myasthenia gravis. Paraneoplastic pure red cell aplasia has also been also reported. Seventy-two percent is Masaoka-Koga stage I at presentation, 22% stage II, and 6% stage III. As in WHO type A disease, stage IV is rare [1]. Overall 5- and 10-year survival is reported 80–100% for stages I and II.

Type B1 thymoma is composed of thymic epithelial cells which are practically indistinguishable from the normal thymus cortex and medulla. A prominent population of immature lymphocytes is present. Like the other types, type B1 thymoma is associated with myasthenia gravis, but additionally hypogammaglobulinemia and pure red cell aplasia have been reported. Invasion in adjacent organs occurs in 12% of patients [11]. Complete surgical resection is possible in 94% of the cases with a recurrence rate of 10%. Ten-year survival rate is >90% [10].

Type B2 thymomas are usually at a more advanced stage. They are predominantly composed of large, polygonal tumor cells in the background of a large population of immature T lymphocytes. The most frequent manifestations (up to 80%) are symptoms arising from myasthenia gravis. Pure red cell aplasia, hypogammaglobulinemia, and other paraneoplastic autoimmune diseases have been described. Up to 53% are stage Masaoka-Koga I or III at presentation, and 8.2% is stage IV. In 5–15% of cases, they are non-resectable, and recurrence rates are 9% after complete resection [10, 12]. Reported 10-year survival rates are between 50 and 100% [1].

Type B3 thymomas are almost always invasive and unresectable at presentation. Like the other types of thymomas, the most frequent association is myasthenia gravis. Pure red cell aplasia and hypogammaglobinemia are rare. The majority of patients are Masaoka-Koga stage II or III at presentation, and stage IV occurs in 20%. Ten-year survival rates range between 50 and 70% [10, 12, 13].

Thymic carcinomas are atypical, invasive epithelial tumors that show resemblance to carcinomas outside the thymus and show a lot of differentiation. Squamous cell carcinomas and undifferentiated carcinomas are the most common subtypes. They are composed of polygonal or round epithelial cells with mild atypia. Invasion of adjacent structures has been reported to occur in 83% of cases. In contrast to thymomas, paraneoplastic syndromes are very rare. Thymic carcinomas have the worst survival rate of the thymic malignancies with only 35% 5-year survival [1, 10, 14].

3. Clinical presentation

Patients with a thymus malignancy can present themselves with complaints due to local compression/invasion or due to a paraneoplastic autoimmune phenomenon, but ~40% of the thymic neoplasms are asymptomatic incidental findings.

Local symptoms are related to the site and size of tumor and compression or invasion on the surrounding tissue. Patients can present themselves with symptoms as chest pain, cough, dysphagia, or stridor. A superior vena cava syndrome can cause swelling of the face and arms and dyspnea. Dyspnea can also be the result of unilateral or bilateral phrenic nerve palsy and pleural or pericardial involvement. The latter can also elicit tachycardia [3]. Systemic symptoms such as fever or weight loss are possible.

3.1 Paraneoplastic autoimmune syndromes

About 40–50% of thymomas are associated with a variety of paraneoplastic autoimmune syndromes, and over 30 associations have been described [1, 15, 16] (**Table 1**). Up to 25% deaths in thymoma are due to the complications of autoimmune syndromes.

The most common paraneoplastic syndrome is myasthenia gravis, followed by pure red cell aplasia and hypogammaglobinemia (Good syndrome).

Ten to twenty percent of patients with myasthenia gravis have a thymoma, and 30–50% of patients with thymoma have myasthenia gravis. It is a neuromuscular disease that leads to varying degrees of muscle weakness. It is caused by autoantibodies that interfere with the acetylcholine receptors in the neuromuscular junction of the voluntary muscles, but the exact mechanism how has yet to be discovered. Systemic symptoms consist of fatigue and general muscle weakness leading to troubles with walking. Myasthenia gravis can antedate the diagnosis of thymoma, be diagnosed concurrently, or occur after thymectomy, with or without recurrence of thymoma [15–17].

Pure red cell aplasia is a profound non-regenerative anemia, characterized by a severe reduction in reticulocytes and absence of erythrocyte precursors in the bone marrow. Five to fifteen percent of patients with thymoma have pure red cell aplasia [16]. It is more common in older women. Remission following surgical excision of the thymoma is uncommon [18].

Neuromuscular diseases	**Myasthenia gravis** Neuromyotonia Rippling muscle disease Polymyositis/dermatomyositis Encephalitis Intestinal pseudo-obstruction
Hematologic autoimmune diseases	Anemia **Pure red cell anemia** Pernicious anemia Hemolytic anemia Aplastic anemia Other isolated cytopenia Immunodeficiencies **Hypogammaglobinemia/Good syndrome** T-cell deficiencies
Dermatologic diseases	Pemphigus Lichen planus Alopecia areata
Endocrine disorders	Addison's disease Cushing's disease Graves' disease
Renal and hepatic disease	Glomerulonephritis Autoimmune hepatitis
Systemic autoimmune diseases	SLE Sjogren's disease Systemic sclerosis **Thymoma-associated multiorgan autoimmunity** (TAMA)

Table 1.
Examples of autoimmune syndromes associated with thymoma.

Patients suffering from hypogammaglobulinemia (or Good syndrome) suffer from recurrent episodes of diarrhea, pulmonary infections, urinary tract infections, and several other bacterial and viral infections. Five percent of patients with Good syndrome have a thymoma, and 10% of patients with a thymoma have hyper-gammaglobulinemia. Thymectomy does not normalize immunoglobulin levels. Treatment consists of administration of intravenous immunoglobulin [16, 19].

Thymoma-associated multiorgan autoimmunity (TAMA) is a severe and often fatal graft-versus-host-like disease that requires special mention. Symptoms are T-cell mediated and cause skin disruptions, liver failure, and diarrhea [3]. Immunoglobulin and methylprednisolone have been described as treatment [20].

4. Diagnostics

4.1 Imaging

Thymic epithelial tumors arise in the anterior mediastinum and are most commonly located between the sternum, the great vessels, and the pericardium. All anterior mediastinal masses should be assessed with a chest computed tomography (CT) with IV contrast [21]. Chest CT can usually show if a thymic tumor is well circumscribed and if invasion in mediastinal fat, the surrounding vessels, or the adjacent lung is present. It can also show the presence of pericardial and/or pleural seeding [16]. Magnetic resonance imaging (MRI) can be used to assess involvement of surrounding tissues [22] and can also be useful to differentiate between thymoma and thymic cysts that demonstrate increased CT attenuation due to hemorrhage or high mucinous content [16]. It can also be considered in patients that cannot tolerate radiocontrast administration.

Thymomas are usually encapsulated, homogenous, and round or oval structures with smooth contours. A cystic component is common. They can range from microscopic size to >30 cm in diameter. Type B thymomas and thymic carcinomas can show calcifications [22]. Thymic carcinomas tend to have irregular borders and necrotic areas and are usually much larger than thymomas. Pleural seeding is seen in both invasive thymoma and thymic carcinoma [23].

Positron-emission tomography (PET) can be useful in the case of thymic carcinoma. Thymic carcinomas have a higher fludeoxyglucose (FDG-18) PET uptake than thymomas. Using a standardized uptake value (SUV) cutoff point of 5.0, thymic carcinoma can be distinguished from thymomas with a sensitivity of 84.6% and a specificity of 92.3%. PET can also be useful for diagnosis of extra thoracic metastases in thymus carcinoma [24].

4.2 Biopsy

When a thymic tumor is considered likely and microscopical complete resection is considered possible, pathological evaluation should be done following surgery. Most thymomas can reliably be identified on the clinical presentation and imaging without the need for a biopsy. Histological classification may be difficult when there is a limited amount of tissue, and invasion in the surrounding tissue cannot be identified on biopsy alone. So even when the diagnosis is uncertain based on clinical presentation and imaging alone, complete surgical resection is advised for both diagnostic and treatment purposes [21].

Historically, it is thought that biopsy can cause pleural seeding. This is the main reason it is recommended to avoid a biopsy when resectable thymoma is suspected [21, 25]. However, there are no known exact data available to describe the proportion of this risk. There are only three case reports published for needle tract implantation of a thymoma reported in the chest wall after biopsy [26–28]. To abstain from a needle biopsy in order to avoid the risk of pleural seeding therefore seems unfounded [29].

In the case of potentially resectable or unresectable disease or when another diagnosis, such as lymphoma, is strongly suspected, tissue diagnosis is necessary. Biopsy should avoid a transpleural approach to prevent tumor seeding in the pleural space [21, 30]. Note that differentiation between lymphoma and thymoma can be difficult when a fine needle aspiration is done, so core needle biopsy or surgical biopsies are preferred [31].

5. Staging

There are several different staging systems for thymoma and thymic carcinoma, but the Masaoka-Koga staging system [32] and the American Joint Committee on Cancer (AJCC) the eighth edition of the TNM prognostic staging system [33] are the most commonly used.

Both staging systems are based on the extent of the primary tumor, invasion of adjacent structures and dissemination. In contrast to other thoracic cancers, both lymph node and distant metastases are considered stage IV disease. The Masaoka-Koga staging system (**Table 2**) is a surgical-pathological system that can only be definitely ascertained after surgery is performed. Historically this has been the most widely used staging system, so most data supporting treatment options is based on patients staged according to the Masaoka-Koga system.

Masaoka-Koga stage	Diagnostic criteria
Stage I	Macroscopically and microscopically completely encapsulated
Stage II	a. Microscopic transcapsular invasion b. Macroscopic invasion into surrounding fatty tissue or grossly adherent to but not through mediastinal pleura or pericardium
Stage III	Macroscopic invasion into neighboring organs (i.e., pericardium, great vessels, lung) a. Without invasion in the great vessels b. With invasion in great vessels
Stage IV	a. Pleural or pericardial dissemination b. Lymphogenous or hematogenous metastases

Table 2.
Masaoka-Koga staging system.

TNM staging AJCC eighth edition			
Primary tumor (T)			
TX	Primary tumor cannot be assessed		
T0	No evidence of primary tumor		
T1	Tumor encapsulated or extending into the mediastinal fat may involve the mediastinal pleura T1a Tumor with no mediastinal pleural involvement T1b tumor with direct invasion of mediastinal pleura		
T2	Tumor with direct invasion of the pericardium (either partial or full thickness)		
T3	Tumor with direct invasion into any of the following: lung, brachiocephalic vein, superior vena cava, phrenic nerve, chest wall, or extrapericardial pulmonary artery or veins		
T4	Tumor with invasion into any of the following: aorta, arch vessels, intrapericardial pulmonary artery, myocardium, or trachea esophagus		
Regional lymph nodes (N)			
NX	Regional lymph nodes cannot be assessed		
N0	No regional lymph node metastases		
N1	Metastases in anterior (perithymic) lymph nodes		
N2	Metastases in deep intrathoracic or cervical lymph nodes		
Distant metastases (M)			
M0	No pleural, pericardial, or distant metastases		
M1	Pleural, pericardial, or distant metastases M1a separate pleural or pericardial nodules M1b pulmonary intraparenchymal nodule or distant organ metastases		
Prognostic stage groups			
	T	N	M
Stage I	T1a,b	N0	M0
Stage II	T2	N0	M0
Stage IIIa	T3	N0	M0
Stage IIIb	T4	N0	M0
Stage IVa	Any T	N1 N0–N1	M0 M1a
Stage IVb	Any T	N2 Any N	M0–M1a M1b

Table 3.
TNM staging AJCC eighth edition.

In 2018, the AJCC published the eighth edition of the TNM staging system (**Table 3**). They incorporated a proposal from the International Association for the Study of Lung Cancer (IASLC) and the International Thymic Malignancy Interest Group (ITMIG) for the staging of thymoma and thymic carcinoma based on the anatomical extend of the tumor combined with prognostic factor. Survival data of 10,808 patients was used [33]. Because of this larger dataset, the addition of nodal metastasis and a better correlation with prognosis, we would advise the AJCC TNM staging system.

6. Management

There are no phase III randomized, clinical trials on the treatment of thymoma and thymic carcinoma. Although they are two different entities, the general management per stage is almost the same. Surgery aimed at complete resection is the cornerstone of thymoma and thymic carcinoma management and should always be pursued.

All patients should be managed by a multidisciplinary team with experience in the management of thymoma and thymic carcinoma. The choice of treatment depends on resectability, stage, and whether or not myasthenia gravis is present. In all stages of thymoma and thymic carcinoma, resectability should be considered. When deemed possible in stages IIIb and IVa, surgery is part of a multimodality approach [25, 34–37].

An example of management according to stage could be as shown in **Table 4**. One should realize though that there is no advise based on phase III randomized controlled trails available and every case should be considered individually and there are different options, as discussed below.

6.1 Treatment thymoma

6.1.1 Resectable disease

Once complete resection of a thymoma is deemed possible, complete resection of the thymus, the tumor, and the invaded structures (including resection of the lung parenchyma or pericardium and vena cava reconstruction if necessary) is

Treatment thymoma and thymic carcinoma according to stage		
AJCC TMN stage	Thymoma	Thymic carcinoma
Stage I	Complete resection	Complete resection
Stage II	Complete resection Consider PORT in WHO type B2/3	Complete resection and PORT
Stage III	**Resectable or potentially resectable disease:** Multimodality approach Consider neoadjuvant chemotherapy in IIIA tumors. Neoadjuvant chemotherapy in IIIb tumors Complete resection or, when not feasible during surgery, maximum debulking PORT **Unresectable disease** Chemoradiation	**Resectable or potentially resectable disease:** Multimodality approach Consider neoadjuvant chemotherapy in IIIA tumors. Neoadjuvant chemotherapy in IIIb tumors Complete resection or, when not feasible during surgery, maximum debulking PORT **Unresectable disease** Chemoradiation
Stage IV	IVA same as stage III IVB chemotherapy or individual approach	IVA same as stage III IVB chemotherapy

Table 4.
Treatment thymoma and thymic carcinoma according to stage.

recommended [21, 25, 34, 36]. Preoperative evaluation for myasthenia gravis is advised. If this is diagnosed, treatment is essential, as myasthenia gravis can cause a postoperative myasthenic crisis or respiratory failure [38]. Thymoma Masaoka-Koga stages I and II have a 5-year survival rate of 100% after surgery [1].

In the case of an incomplete resection, postoperative radiotherapy (PORT), either on the primary tumor or on isolated metastasis, is recommended to reduce the risk of recurrence [35, 39]. In the past PORT was considered standard treatment for stage II completely resected tumors [7, 40]. Nowadays PORT in completely resected stages I and II WHO type A, AB, and B1 thymoma is not considered useful [10, 41–43]. Because of a high recurrence rate (even after R0 resection) PORT is advised for the higher stages and for WHO-type B2/3 thymoma and thymic carcinoma [21, 44], although the data are somewhat conflicting in this [7].

6.1.2 Potentially resectable disease

More extensive thymomas can be initially irresectable but potentially resectable after neoadjuvant treatment. A multimodality approach containing neoadjuvant chemotherapy with or without postoperative radiotherapy should be used, depending on WHO type and resection margins [21, 35, 45–47].

Potential advantages of neoadjuvant chemotherapy are tumor downstaging and increasing the likelihood of complete resection. However, because the available data on chemotherapy in thymoma is based on small, phase II studies, there is no optimal chemotherapeutic regime established [21]. Potential disadvantages could be complications due to chemotherapy and longer operating time [48]. There is even some recent data suggesting that there is no overall survival benefit to be expected from neoadjuvant chemotherapy before surgery [48–50]. In the cases of extensive pleural disease, several institutions have reported small series of extrapleural pneumonectomy for stage IVA disease with excellent outcomes and low morbidity [51].

There are no RCT's available to settle this matter. For now, it is recommended to use neoadjuvant chemotherapy to downstage unresectable thymic malignancies before surgery [21]. Obviously, reevaluation after neoadjuvant therapy to determine whether or not the tumor responded sufficiently is mandatory. There is evidence supporting maximum debulking, combined with PORT and/or adjuvant chemotherapy, to benefit survival from a thymoma which turns out to be unresectable during surgery. This is, however, based on retrospective data, so selection bias could cloud this positive outcome [3, 52].

6.1.3 Unresectable disease

In the case of unresectable disease or the patients is inoperable due to condition or comorbidity, the possibility of radiation therapy should be assessed. If radiation is feasible, concurrent chemoradiation is advised. If radiation is not possible due to a too large field, palliative chemotherapy is recommended. But even in that setting, long-term disease control and survival can be sometimes pursued, and even a combination of radiation on the primary tumor combined with resection of metastasis could be considered [21].

Chemotherapy is the primary modality in systemic management of unresectable thymoma. Thymomas are known to be sensitive to chemotherapy, possible due to a "lymphocytic effect" of cytotoxic agents. Due to the rarity of the disease and surgery with or without PORT being the cornerstone of treatment, there are no randomized controlled trails available to select a preferred regime. Platinum-based combinations are standard of care, the most popular regimes being cisplatin with anthracycline and/or etoposide. The response rate range of these regimens is between 25 and 100% [53]. The preferred regime by the NCCN is cisplatin/doxorubicin/cyclophosphamide [21, 54].

Stereotactic radiotherapy (SBRT) may be appropriate for limited focal metastasis; conventional fractionation is appropriate for larger metastasis [21].

Response rates for second-line therapy range from 15 to 39% [55]. Pemetrexed and paclitaxel are considered the most efficacious in second-line treatment of thymic malignancies, although this is based on small phase II studies and expert opinion [21, 56, 57].

Checkpoint inhibitors. Programmed death ligand 1 (PD-L1) expression is high (82%) in thymoma, especially in WHO type B thymoma [58]. Even so, based on a phase II study on pembrolizumab (a humanized IgG4 antibody to PD-L1) in 33 thymic epithelial tumors (including 7 thymomas), immunotherapy is not recommended in thymoma. This is because of the high grade of immune-related events that was shown in seven thymoma patients during this study; 71% had grade 3 or higher immune-related adverse events (including myocarditis) [59]. Avelumab is a fully human IgG1 anti-PD-L1 antibody that showed less adverse events (38%) in a phase I trial (n = 7). However, it is currently under clinical development, and no phase II data is available [60].

The high rate of immune-related side effect was expected; the physiological role of the thymus is to induce tolerance to self-antigens and deletion of autoimmune T cells. In the normal thymus, PD-1/PL-D1 expression regulates this self-tolerant T-cell repertoire. It is thought that disruption of the PD-1/PDL-1 system could lead to significant alteration of the T-cell population and therefore cause autoimmune-related adverse events in the case of checkpoint inhibition [61].

Targeted therapies. Although there is high epidermal growth factor receptor (EGFR) expression in immunohistochemical staining of thymic epithelial tumors (71% for thymoma and 53% for thymic carcinoma), there is no correlation between the EGFR status and EGFR mutations. Experience with targeted therapies in thymoma is very limited and based on a small number of heterogenic phase II studies, but as for now this shows that there is no place for EGFR inhibitors in the treatment of thymoma and thymic carcinoma [7]. KIT-inhibition (inhibition of a transmembrane type III tyrosine kinase receptor) may show some promises in thymic carcinomas, but as thymomas do not show c-KIT expression [62], KIT-inhibition is not effective. There is some phase II experience in insulin-like growth factor (IGFR) inhibitors in thymoma patients that have shown some promising results [63]. Octreotide (a somatostatin analog) plus prednisolone may be useful in patients who have a positive octreotide scan [64].

6.1.4 *Recurrent disease*

The recurrence rate of thymoma after complete resection is 10–30%, and this can occur many years after initial treatment. Surgical resection of recurrent disease can be associated with long-term survival and should be considered for patients with recurrent thymoma. In pleural "drop" lesions, repeated resection is considered safe [50, 65].

6.2 Treatment thymic carcinoma

Similar to thymoma, surgery aimed at complete resection is the cornerstone of thymic carcinoma treatment, and the principles of first-line treatment in resectable disease are more or less the same. Five-year survival rate of 100% is reported for completely resected stage I disease going down to 17% in stage IVb disease [66]. Patients with a thymic carcinoma have a high risk of recurrent disease. Therefore, some centers offer PORT (with or without chemotherapy) regardless of stage and resection margins [3, 21]. The available data is yet again limited, and there are indications that adjuvant therapy is not beneficial in R0-resected stage I thymic carcinoma [21, 42, 67].

Chemotherapy. Thymic carcinomas respond less to chemotherapy than thymomas. Carboplatin/paclitaxel has the highest response rate in patients with thymic carcinoma, but even so this is only 22–36% [21, 55]. Response rates for second-line chemotherapy in thymic carcinoma are even worse (4–12%) [55].

Checkpoint inhibitors. Second-line treatment with pembrolizumab showed promising results in a phase II trial containing 40 patients with thymic carcinoma. There was an ORR of 22.5%, and the median duration of response was 22 months. While less in thymomas, there was still a high rate of immune-related adverse events (15%), including two cases of severe myocarditis [59]. A recently published study on nivolumab in thymic carcinoma patients showed no objective response in 15 patients, although 5 patients showed stable disease for more than 24 weeks [68].

Targeted therapies. The same as in thymoma, experience with targeted therapies in thymoma is very limited and based on small phase II studies and individual case reports. Sunitinib may be beneficial for patients with a c-KIT mutation, although the mutation rate is rare <10% [10, 69]. IGFR inhibition and octreotide did not show any activity in thymic carcinoma, in contrast to thymomas [63, 64].

6.3 Follow-up

After primary resection, expert opinion on follow-up consists of a CT scan every 6 months for 2 years, then annually for 5 years for thymic carcinoma and annually for 10 years for thymomas [21], although an exceptional case of late recurrence has been reported [70].

7. Conclusion

Thymomas and thymic carcinomas are rare mediastinal tumors, and although the course of a thymoma can be indolent, they can indeed be locally invasive and metastasize. Thymic carcinomas more often are disseminated at presentation. Therefore, both are considered malignant. Forty to fifty percent of thymomas are related to autoimmune paraneoplastic syndromes, the most common being myasthenia gravis. Resection of the thymus can also act as treatment for the paraneoplastic syndrome. However, thymic treatment does not always resolve those paraneoplastic syndromes.

Because of the improved representation of the N-stage and correlation to prognosis, rather than surgical resectability, we recommend the AJCC eighth TMN classification.

There is no phase III data available on the management of thymic epithelial tumors. Surgery is considered the cornerstone of thymoma and thymic carcinoma management in resectable disease and even in recurrent disease. Neoadjuvant treatment and PORT should be considered according to stage.

In metastatic disease chemotherapy containing an anthracycline is advised. For recurrent metastatic disease sunitinib and octreotide, among other things, could be considered. A special note on checkpoint inhibitors should be made. Although they do show promising results in thymic carcinoma, the rate of immune-related adverse events is too high to consider this a valuable option for the treatment of thymoma right now.

The lack of phase III level evidence due to the rarity of the disease calls for collaboration in research to improve the quality and impact of thymic malignancy treatment. Such efforts are currently underway, and hopefully this will lead to better and more treatment options in the future.

Author details

Annette Rebecca Bijsmans and Robin Cornelissen*
Erasmus MC Cancer Institute, Rotterdam, The Netherlands

*Address all correspondence to: r.cornelissen@erasmusmc.nl

References

[1] Takanaka T, Ishida T, Handa Y, Tsutsui S, Matsuda H. Ectopic thymoma presenting as a giant intrathoracic mass: A case report. Journal of Cardiothoracic Surgery. 2012

[2] Tazelaar HD, Roden AC. Pathology of Mediastinal Tumors. UptoDate.com. [Online]. [Zugriff am April, 2019]

[3] Travis WD, Brambilla E, Müller-Hermelink HK, Harris CC. Pathology & Genetics Tumours of the Lung, Pleura. Lyon: IARC Press; 2004. pp. 145-247

[4] "Thymoma and thymic Carcinomas NCCN Evidence Blocks," National Comprehensive Cancer Network guidelines, 1 March 2019. [Online]. Available: https://www.nccn.org/professionals/physician_gls/pdf/thymic_blocks.pdf [Accessed: 1 April 2019]

[5] Ströbel P, Bauwer A, Puppe B, Kraushaar T, Krein A, Toyka K, et al. Tumor recurrence and survival in patients treated for thymomas and thymic squamous cell carcinomas: A retrospective analysis. Journal of Clinical Oncology. 2004;**22**(8):1501-1509

[6] Amin AB, Edge S, Greene F, Byrd DR, Brookland RK, Washinton MK, et al. AJCC (American Joint Committee on Cancer) Cancer Staging Manual. 8th ed. Chicago: Springer; 2017

[7] Awad WI, Symmans PJ, Dussek JE. Recurrence of stage I thymoma 32 years after total excision. The Annals of Thoracic Surgery. 1998;**66**(6):2106-2108

[8] Berghmans T, Durieux V, Holbrechts S, Jungels C, Lafitte JJ, Meert AP, et al. Systemic treatments for thymoma and thymic carcinoma: A systematic review. Lung Cancer. 2018;**126**:25-31. [Epub ahead of print]

[9] Bernard C, Frith H, Pasquet F, Kerever S, Jamillioux Y, Tronc F, et al. Thymoma associated with autoimmune diseases: 85 cases and literature review. Autoimmunity Reviews. 2016;**15**(1):82-92

[10] Bretti S, Berrutti A, Loddo C, Sperone P, Casadio C, Tessa M, et al. Multimodal management of stages III-IVa malignant thymoma. Lung Cancer. 2004;**44**(1):69-77

[11] Cata JP, Lasala JD, Williams W, Mena GE. Myasthenia gravis and thymoma surgery: A clinical update for the cardiothoracic anesthesiologist. Journal of Cardiothoracic and Vascular Anesthesia. 2018;**2018**. [Epub ahead of print]

[12] Cavelcante P, Marcuzzo S, Franzi S, Galbardi B, Maggi L, Motta T, et al. Epstein-Barr virus in tumor-infiltrating B cells of myasthenia gravis thymoma: an innocent bystander or an autoimmunity mediator? Oncotarget. 2017;**8**:95432-95449

[13] Cho J, Kim HS, Ku BM, Choi YL, Cristescu R, Han J, et al. Pembrolizumab for patients with refractory or relapsed thymic epithelial tumor: An open-label Phase II trial. Journal of Clinical Oncology. 2018. [Epub ahead of print]

[14] Detterbeck F, Youssef S, Ruffini E, Okumura M. A review of prognostic factors in thymic malignancies. Journal of Thoracic Oncology. 2011;**7**(Suppl 3):S1698-S1704

[15] Detterbeck FC. Evaluation and Treatment of Stage I and II Thymoma. Journal of Thoracic Oncology. 2010;**10**(Suppl 4):S318-S322

[16] Detterbeck FC, Parsons AM. Management of stage I and II thymoma. Thoracic Surgery Clinics. 2011;**21**(1):59-67

[17] Forguer JA, Rong N, Fakiris AJ, Loehrer PJ, Johnstone PA. Postoperative radiotherapy after surgical resection of thymoma: Differing roles in localized and regional disease. International Journal of Radiation Oncology, Biology, Physics. 2010;**76**(2):440-445

[18] Fujiwara K, Matsumura A, Tanaka H, Ohmori K, Yamamoto S, Iuchi K. Needle tract implantation of thymoma after transthoracic needle biopsy. Kyobu Geka. 2003;**56**(6):448-451

[19] Furie B, Atkins MB, Mayer RJ, Cassileth PA. Clinical Hematology and Oncology: Presentation, Diagnosis and Treatment. London, Churchill Livingstone: Elsevier Health Science; 2003

[20] Gbolahan OB, Porter RF, Salter JT, Yiannoutsos C, Burns M, Chiorean EG, et al. A Phase II study of pemetrexed in patients with recurrent thymoma and thymic carcinoma. Journal of Thoracic Oncology. 2018;**13**(12):1940-1948

[21] Girard N. Thymic malignancies: Twisting between autoimmunity and immunotherapy. Lung Cancer. 2017;**110**:68-70

[22] Guleria P, Huisain N, Shukla S, Kumar S, Pershad R, Jain D. PD-L1 immuno-expression assay in thymomas: Study of 84 cases and review of literature. Annals of Diagnostic Pathology. 2018;**34**:135-141

[23] Hamaji M, Ali SO, Burt BM. A meta-analysis of induction therapy for advanced thymic epithelial tumors. The Annals of Thoracic Surgery. 2015;**99**(5):1848-1856

[24] Hamaji M, Shah RM, Ali SO, Bettenhaussen A, Lee HS, Burt BM. A meta-analysis of postoperative radiotherapy for thymic carcinoma. The Annals of Thoracic Surgery. 2017;**103**(5):1668-1675

[25] Hamaji M, Kojima F, Omasa M, Sozu T, Sato T, Chen F, et al. A meta-analysis of debulking surgery versus surgical biopsy for unresectable thymoma. European Journal of Cardio-Thoracic Surgery. 2015;**47**(4):602-607

[26] Hirokawa M, Sawada K, Fuijshima N, Nakao S, Urabe A, Dan K, et al. Long-term response and outcome following immunosuppressive therapy in thymoma-associated pure red cell aplasia: a nationwide cohort study in Japan by the PRCA collaborative study group. Haematologica. 2008;**93**(1):27-33

[27] Jung JI, Kim HH, Park SH, Lee YS. Malignant ectopic thymoma in the neck: A case report. AJNR. American Journal of Neuroradiology. 1999;**20**(9):1747-1749

[28] Kanzaki R, Kanou T, Ose N, Funaki S, Shintani Y, Minami M, et al. Long-term outcomes of advanced thymoma in patients undergoing preoperative chemotherapy or chemoradiotherapy followed by surgery: A 20-year experience. Interactive Cardiovascular and Thoracic Surgery. 2019;**28**(3):360-367

[29] Katsuya Y, Horinouchi H, Seto T, Umemura S, Hosomi Y, Satouchi M, et al. Single-arm, multicentre, phase II trial of nivolumab for unresectable or recurrent thymic carcinoma: PRIMER study. European Journal of Cancer. 2019;**113**:78-86

[30] Kattach H, Hasan S, Clelland C, Pillai R. Seeding of stage I thymoma into the chest wall 12 years after needle biopsy. The Annals of Thoracic Surgery. 2005;**79**(1):323-324

[31] Kim ES, Putnam JB, Komaki R, Walsh GL, Ro JY, Shin HJ, et al. Phase II study of a multidisciplinary approach with induction chemotherapy, followed by surgical resection, radiation therapy, and consolidation chemotherapy for unresectable malignant thymomas:

Final report. Lung Cancer. 2004;**44**(3):369-379

[32] Kondo K, Yoshizawa K, Tsuyuguchi M, Kimura S, Sumitomo M, Morita J, et al. WHO histologic classification is a prognostic indicator in thymoma. The Annals of Thoracic Surgery. 2004;**77**(4):1183-1188

[33] Lemma GL, Lee JW, Aisner SC, Langer CJ, Tester WJ, Johnson DH, et al. Phase II study of carboplatin and paclitaxel in advanced thymoma and thymic carcinoma. Journal of Clinical Oncology. 2011;**29**(15):2060-2065

[34] Lewis JE, Wick MR, Scheithauwer BW, Bernatz PE, Taylor WF. Thymoma. A clinicopathologic review. Cancer. 1987;**60**(11):2727-2743

[35] Litvak AM, Woo K, Hayes S, Huang J, Rimner A, Sima CS, et al. Clinical characteristics and outcomes for patients with thymic carcinoma: evaluation of Masaoka staging. Journal of Thoracic Oncology. 2014;**9**(12):1810-1815

[36] Loeher PJ, Wang W, Johnson DH, Aisner SC, Ettiniger DS. Eastern Cooperative Oncology Group Phase II Trial. Journal of Clinical Oncology. 2004;**22**(2):293-299

[37] Loeher PJ, Kim K, Aisner SC, Livingston R, Einhorn LH, Johnson D, et al. Cisplatin plus doxorubicin plus cyclophosphamide in metastatic or recurrent thymoma: Final results of an intergroup trial. The Eastern Cooperative Oncology Group, Southwest Oncology Group, and Southeastern Cancer Study Group. Journal of Clinical Oncology. 1994;**12**(6):1164-1168

[38] Lucchi M, Davini F, Ricciardi R, Duranti L, Boldrini L, Palmiero G, et al. Management of pleural recurrence after curative resection of thymoma. The Journal of Thoracic and Cardiovascular Surgery. 2009;**137**(5):1185-1189

[39] Marom EM. Imaging thymoma. Journal of Thoracic Oncology. 2010;**5**(10-Suppl 4):S296-S303

[40] Masaoka A. Staging system of thymoma. Journal of Thoracic Oncology. 2010;**5**(10 suppl 4):S304-S312

[41] Mehran R, Ghosh R, Maziak D, O'Rourke K, Shamji F. Surgical treatment of thymoma. Canadian Journal of Surgery. 2002;**45**(1):25-30

[42] Meneshian A, Giaccone G, Olivier KR. Clinical presentation and management of thymoma and thymic carcinoma. UptoDate.com, 4 April 2019. [Online]. [Accessed: April 2019]

[43] Merveilleux du Vignaux C, Dansin E, Mhanna L, Greillier L, Pinchon E, Kerjouan M, et al. Systemic therapy in advanced thymic epithelial tumors: Insights from the rythmic prospective cohort. Journal of Thoracic Oncology. 2018;**13**(11):1762-1770

[44] Morrissey B, Adams H, Gibbs AR, Crane MD. Percutaneous needle biopsy of the mediastinum: Review of 94 procedures. Thorax. 1993;**48**(6):632-637

[45] Nagasaka T, Nakashima N, Nunome H. Needle tract implantation of thymoma after transthoracic needle biopsy. Journal of Clinical Pathology. 1993;**46**(3):278-279

[46] Nakahara K, Ogno K, Hashimoto J, Maeda H, Miyoshi S, Sakurai M, et al. Thymoma: Results with complete resection and adjuvant postoperative irradiation in 141 consecutive patients. The Journal of Thoracic and Cardiovascular Surgery. 1988;**95**(6):1041-1047

[47] Nishino M, Ashiku SK, Kocher ON, Thurer RL, Bioselle PM, Hatabu H. The thymus: A comprehensive review. Radiographics. 2006;**26**(2):335-348

[48] Okereke IC, Kesler KA, Freeman RK, Rieger KM, Birdas TJ, Ascioti AJ, et al. Thymic carcinoma: Outcomes after surgical resection. The Annals of Thoracic Surgery. 2012;**93**(5):1668-1672

[49] Okumura M, Ohta M, Tateyama H, Nakagawa K, Matsumura A, Maeda H, et al. The World Health Organization histologic classification system reflects the oncologic behavior of thymoma: a clinical study of 273 patients. Cancer. 2002;**94**(3):624-632

[50] Omasa M, Date H, Sozu T, Sato T, Nagai K, Yokoi K, et al. Postoperative radiotherapy is effective for thymic carcinoma but not for thymoma in stage II and III thymic epithelial tumors: The Japanese Association for Research on the Thymus Database Study. Cancer. 2015;**121**(7):1008-1016

[51] Park S, Park IK, Kim YT, Lee GD, Kim DK, Cho JH, et al. Comparison of neoadjuvant chemotherapy followed by surgery to upfront surgery for thymic malignancy. The Annals of Thoracic Surgery. 2019;**107**(2):355-362

[52] Rajan A, Carter CA, Berman A, Cao L, Kelly RJ, Thomas A, et al. Cixutumumab for patients with recurrent or refractory advanced thymic epithelial tumours: A multicentre, open-label, phase 2 trial. The Lancet Oncology. 2014;**15**(2):191-200

[53] Rajan A, Heery C, Mamman A, Pittaluga S, Lepone L, Donahue R, et al. OA18.03 safety and clinical activity of avelumab (MSB0010718C; Anti-PD-L1) in patients with advanced thymic epithelial tumors (TETs). Journal of Thoracic Oncology. 2017;**12**(1):S314-S315

[54] Ried M, Potzger T, Sziklavari Z, Diez C, Neu R, Schalke B, et al. Extended surgical resections of advanced thymoma Masaoka stages III and IVa facilitate outcome. The Thoracic and Cardiovascular Surgeon. 2014;**62**(2):161-168

[55] Riely GJ, Huang J. Induction therapy for locally advanced thymoma. Journal of Thoracic Oncology. 2010;**5** (10 suppl 4):S323-S326

[56] Rimner A, Yao X, Huang J, Antonicelli A, Amhad U, Korts RJ, et al. Postoperative radiation therapy is associated with longer overall survival in completely resected Stage II and III thymoma-an analysis of the international thymic malignancies interest group retrospective database. Journal of Thoracic Oncology. 2016;**11**(10):1785-1792

[57] Sasaki M, Kuwabara Y, Ichiya Y, Akashi Y, Yoshida T, Nakagawa M, et al. Differential diagnosis of thymic tumors using a combination of 11C-methionine PET and FDG PET. Journal of Nuclear Medicine. 1999;**40**(10):1595-1601

[58] Scorsetti M, Leo F, Trama A, D'Angelillo R, Serpico D, Macereli M, et al. Thymoma and thymic carcinomas. Critical Reviews in Oncology/Hematology. 2016;**99**:332-350

[59] Siesling S, van der Zwan JM, Izarzugaza I, Jaal J, Treasure T, Foschi R, et al. Rare thoracic cancers, including peritoneum mesothelioma. European Journal of Cancer. 2012;**48**(7):949-960

[60] Ströbel P, Hohenberger P, Marx A. Thymoma and thymic carcinoma: Molecular pathology and targeted therapy. Journal of Thoracic Oncology. 2010;**5**(10 suppl 4):S286-S290

[61] Tarr PE, Sneller MC, Mechanic LJ, Economides A, Egar CM, Strober W, et al. Infections in patients with immunodeficiency with thymoma (Good syndrome). Report of 5 cases and review of the literature. Medicine. 2001;**80**(2):123-133

[62] Teh BT, McArdle J, Chan SP, Menon J, Hartley L, Pullan P, et al. Clinicopathologic studies of thymic carcinoids in multiple endocrine

neoplasia type 1. Medicine (Baltimore). 1997;**76**(1):21-29

[63] Thomas A, Rajan A, Berman A, Giaccone G. Multiorgan autoimmune manifestations associated with thymoma. Journal of Thoracic Oncology. 2015;**10**(2):e5-e7

[64] Thomas A, Rajan A, Beran A, Tomita Y, Brzezniak C, Lee MJ, et al. Sunitinib in patients with chemotherapy-refractory thymoma and thymic carcinoma: An open-label phase 2 trial. The Lancet Oncology. 2015;**16**(2):177-186

[65] Tomiyoma N, Johkoh T, Mihara N, Honda O, Kozuka T, Koyama M, et al. Using the World Health Organization Classification of thymic epithelial neoplasms to describe CT findings. AJR. American Journal of Roentgenology. 2002;**179**(4):881-886

[66] Travis WD, Brambilla E, Müller-Hermelink HK, Harris CC. Pathology & Genetics Tumours of the Lung, Pleura, Thymus and Heart. lyon: IARC Press; 2004. pp. 145-247

[67] Wei Y, Gu Z, Shen Y, Fu J, Tan L, Zhang P, et al. Preoperative induction therapy for locally advanced thymic tumors: A retrospective analysis using the ChART database. Journal of Thoracic Disease. 2016;**8**(4):665-672

[68] Willcox N, Leite MI, Kadota Y, Jones M, Meager A, Subrahmanyam P, et al. Autoimmunizing mechanisms in thymoma and thymus. Annals of the New York Academy of Sciences. 2008;**1132**(1):163-172

[69] Wright CD. Extended resections for thymic malignancies. Journal of Thoracic Oncology. 2010;**10**(supp 4):S344-S347

[70] Wright CD. Pleuropneumonectomy for the treatment of Masaoka stage IVA thymoma. The Annals of Thoracic Surgery. 2006;**82**(4):1234-1239

Chapter 8

Clinical Presentation of Myasthenia Gravis

Jianu Catalin, Jianu Silviana and Barsan Claudia

Abstract

Despite advances in applied sciences, myasthenia gravis (MG) remains a challenging disorder to diagnose and treat. The clinical presentation results in either transient or persistent painless weakness and abnormal fatigability of any (ocular, bulbar, limbs, trunk, respiratory) or all voluntary (skeletal) muscles; however, it is usually not to the same extent. Several scoring systems of MG signs or the global state of the patient have been proposed in an attempt to provide a standard scheme for use by all investigators. Some patients may have non-muscle-related complaints due to different disorders which may be associated with MG (thymoma, thyroid disorders, other autoimmune diseases, etc.).

Keywords: myasthenia gravis, transient or persistent weakness, skeletal muscles, thymoma

1. Myasthenia gravis: overview

Myasthenia gravis (MG) is a neuromuscular autoimmune disease characterized by the production of autoantibodies directed against molecules involved in neuromuscular transmission (NMT): the $\alpha1$ subunit of the nicotinic postsynaptic acetylcholine receptors (AChR) and muscle-specific tyrosine kinase (MuSK) [1–3].

MG occurs more frequently in women than men; the age of onset in women is in their second and third decade of life, while in men, it is in the fourth [1, 4]. Moreover, there is a second peak of incidence in the sixth and seventh decades, with men being more affected. Epidemiologically, it was found that men tend to experience more severe symptoms [4, 5].

Clinically, MG is defined by a painless, fluctuant muscle weakness that progressively increases with repetitive muscle action but decreases with rest [1–3]. The degree of weakness is dependent on the exertion of the skeletal muscle group involved, but in some cases, it may change over longer periods without any evident cause [6].

Even though all types of voluntary muscle can be involved during the disease course, MG characteristically begins with a few isolated signs and spreads to other muscles within a variable period of time (weeks, months, or even years) [6].

In about 15–20% of the patients, myasthenic symptoms remain confined to the ocular muscles; however, with disease progression and usually within 2 years, the rest of them develop bulbar symptoms (i.e., dysphagia, dysarthria) and facial, axial, and limb weakness [1, 2, 6, 7].

The maximum severity of MG manifestations is usually reported during the first year in two-thirds of patients [1]. Additionally, it has become evident that, in general, the illness tends to stabilize, improve (57%), or even resolve (13%) after several years [3, 6].

It is important to emphasize that in MG, symptoms may worsen in certain conditions including stress, systemic illness (especially upper respiratory infections), hypo−/hyperthyroidism, pregnancy, menstrual cycle, exposure to heat, operative procedures, drugs affecting NMT, and fever [1, 5, 8]. However, in the majority of cases, no precipitating factor can be found [3, 5]. A severe exacerbation requiring endotracheal intubation with mechanical ventilation is defined as myasthenic crisis (Class V myasthenia by MG Foundation of America) [5].

The treatment used in MG includes symptomatic treatment (acetylcholinesterase inhibitors), rapid short-term immunomodulating therapies (plasmapheresis and intravenous immunoglobulin), chronic long-term immunomodulating treatment (glucocorticoids and/or other immunosuppressive agents), and, in selected patients, surgical treatment (thymectomy). In all cases, MG management should be individualized according to patient characteristics and the severity of the disease [3].

Currently, the mortality of MG is extremely low, considering that only among the 19% of the patients with severe generalized MG also need endotracheal intubation; the mortality can reach 8% despite ventilation [5, 6, 9].

2. Clinical features

The cardinal features of the initial course of MG are the transient or persistent weakness and abnormal fatigability of skeletal muscles that are typically least severe in the morning and after rest and worst as the day progresses and after repetitive activities [1, 3, 5] (**Table 1**).

The weakness, which is mostly asymmetrical, specifically affects the extraocular, bulbar, and proximal limb or truncal musculature and, in more rare cases, the respiratory muscles [3–5].

In about two-thirds of the patients with MG, the presenting symptoms are unilateral or asymmetrical ptosis and/or diplopia due to the involvement of extrinsic ocular muscles [2–4].

Over 15% of patients show (as an initial MG symptom) bulbar weakness, leading to slurred or nasal speech, voice alterations, or difficulty in chewing or swallowing; neck and extremity weaknesses are flagged as complaints in about 5% of patients [2, 5, 7, 10].

Importantly, careful questioning frequently reveals evidence of earlier subtle myasthenic manifestations, such as repeated purchases of eyeglasses to correct blurred vision or avoidance of foods that became difficult to chew or swallow. Also, family members may observe a changed, sleepy or sad, facial appearance caused by ptosis or facial weakness [1].

It has to be mentioned that, in MG, cognition, coordination, and tendon reflexes are normal. Also, local muscle atrophy is rarely seen in myasthenic patients, being reported especially in MuSK-antibody MG patients [1, 2, 5, 6].

2.1 Ocular symptoms

Ocular symptoms are the most frequent manifestations of MG, ultimately being present in 90% of patients [6]. The major ocular symptoms associated with MG are

Level	Symptoms	Early onset <40 years	Late onset >40 years	Thymoma
Ocular muscles	• Diplopia	++	++	+/−
	• Ptosis	++	+	+/−
Bulbar muscles	• Articulation	++	+/−	+/−
	• Face	+	+/−	+/−
	• Chewing	+/−	+/−	+/−
	• Swallowing	+/−	+/−	+/−
	• Neck	+/−	+/−	+/−
Limbs muscles	• -Arms	+	+/−	+/−
	• -Hands and fingers	+	+/−	+/−
	• -Legs	++	+/−	+/−
Generalized	+/−	+/−	+/−	+
Respiration	+/−	+/−	+/−	+/−

Table 1.
Clinical manifestations of myasthenia gravis.

fluctuating ptosis (often with compensatory wrinkling of the forehead), diplopia, and, in milder cases, blurry vision [3, 5]. These manifestations may be intermittent in the early stages, typically becoming worse in the evening, while reading or driving, and especially in bright sunlight [1].

In MG a certain degree of photophobia is seen, commonly worsening the ptosis and/or diplopia; as a consequence, some patients often choose to wear dark sunglasses [1, 3].

Weakness involving one or more ocular muscles is, by definition, asymmetric, fluctuating, and fatigable [1]. The most frequently affected extraocular muscle is the medial rectus [3]. Furthermore, in MG, the pattern of weakness cannot be correlated with lesions of one or more nerves, and the pupillary responses are normal [1].

Asymmetric ptosis of the alternating sides over time is considered pathognomonic of MG. In some cases, ptosis can be severe enough to totally occlude vision if it is bilateral [1, 3].

Weakness of the orbicularis oculi muscles, frequently seen in MG patients, leads to incomplete closure of the eyelids, which produces discomfort by allowing soap or water in the eyes during bathing [1, 5]. It should also be mentioned that the weakness of lateral and medial recti can determine a pseudo-internuclear ophthalmoplegia with limited adduction of one eye and nystagmus of the abducting contralateral eye [5].

2.2 Bulbar symptoms

In about 15% of patients [11] with MG, bulbar symptoms, generally manifested as oropharyngeal muscle weakness, are evident from the beginning [12]; during the course of the disease, bulbar muscle involvement can be found in 60% of patients [3]. The characteristic bulbar symptoms seen in MG include fatigable chewing (particularly solid food) and swallowing (particularly liquids), dysarthria, and inadequate maintenance of the upper airway. Typically, the time needed for eating a meal increases, and conversation becomes difficult, especially while eating [1, 3, 6].

Dysarthria: Speech difficulties manifesting as dysarthria and nasality are commonly seen in MG. Initially, dysarthria is an isolated and fluctuating symptom that occurs mostly under the influence of emotions, worsens with prolonged talking, and disappears after a "silent period" [6]. Weakness of laryngeal muscles causes hoarseness; the voice may become weaker in volume, but MG does not determine aphonia [1, 6]. Orbicularis oris weakness is usually observed as the patient becomes unable to whistle, to kiss, and to blow up a balloon or by difficulty in pronouncing certain letters (p, f, s). Importantly, vocal cord paralysis, leading to stridor, or "crowing" during attempted deep inspirations, may be a sign of severe respiratory distress requiring endotracheal intubation [5, 6].

Dysphagia in MG is caused by weakness of the lips, the tongue, the masseter, and the pharyngeal muscles or sometimes a combination of these [6]. Dysphagia found in MG patients is typically associated with several characteristic signs as follows: difficulty chewing caused by incomplete jaw closure resulting from masseter and temporalis muscle weakness; difficulty swallowing exposing the patient to a high risk of aspiration, leading to coughing or choking especially while drinking; nasal regurgitation of liquids due to palatal muscle weakness; sensation that food is sticking in the throat as a consequence of upper pharyngeal muscle weakness; and weight loss—which can be correlated with the severity of eating difficulties. It is important to emphasize that dysphagia can precipitate a myasthenic crisis in patients with MG [1, 5, 6].

2.3 Facial appearance

Myasthenic patients usually have a facial appearance that gives the impression of a sleepy, expressionless, or sad person. This particular appearance is caused mostly by ptosis and facial weakness. Classical features found in MG are also the "myasthenic snarl" and the "rire vertical." These signs occur as attempting to smile produce contraction of the medial part of the upper lip and a horizontal contraction of the corners of the mouth with loss of the natural upward curling and thus, gives the patient's smile the appearance of a sneer. The weakness of the facial muscles usually occurs insidiously and can be asymmetric. Sometimes, a chronic contracted frontalis muscle may give a worried or surprised look to the patient. If weakness is severe, the jaw will tend to hang open and determine the patient to actively hold the mouth closed by sitting with a hand on the chin for support (studious or attentive appearance) [1, 6].

2.4 Limb, trunk, and respiratory weakness

Any trunk or limb muscle may be involved, but some are more often affected than are others; thus, neck flexors are weaker than neck extensors, and the deltoids, triceps, and extensors of the wrist and fingers and ankle dorsiflexors are usually more affected than other limb muscles. MG limb weakness is mostly proximal and often asymmetric [1, 5]. In MG the arms are typically more affected than the legs; also, in the upper extremities, the extensors are often involved before the flexors, while in the lower extremities, the reverse usually occurs [3, 5].

The main complains of the patients with MG which present weakness of the limbs or trunk muscles include fatigability, unexplained feelings of heaviness, inability to maintain arms at a higher position for a long period of time (i.e., when hanging laundry or washing hair), and difficulty in going up and down the stairs [6].

In some cases, severe weakness of neck extensor muscles leads to difficulty in balancing the head sometimes producing a "dropped head syndrome." Pain in the back and girdle muscles is frequently reported as a natural consequence of the insufficiency of the postural muscles; however, MG is typically not associated with chronic pain [1, 3, 5, 6].

Respiratory muscle weakness is revealed by limited chest wall movement and manifest use of accessory muscles of respiration. An important diaphragmatic weakness leads to orthopnea compromising the respiratory efficiency when the patient lies supine [4]. Respiratory muscle weakness may cause life-threatening myasthenic crisis with acute respiratory failure requiring immediate intubation, mechanical ventilation, and nasogastric tube feeding [3].

Note: MG is more frequently associated with other autoimmune disease than the general population. Among the autoimmune conditions found in MG patients are hyperthyroidism, rheumatoid arthritis, scleroderma, ulcerative colitis, pernicious anemia, Sjogren's syndrome, and sarcoidosis. Also, autonomic neuropathies, inflammatory myopathies, various autoimmune channelopathies, or acquired neuromyotonia (Isaac's syndrome) may be seen in patients with MG especially if associated with thymoma. Importantly, in MG patients with tachycardia or exophthalmos, a possible hyperthyroidism should always be addressed; it has to be mentioned that, in these cases, weakness may persist despite adequate management of MG [6, 13].

3. Physical examination

The physical examination should detect fatigable weakness in specific muscle groups by repetitive or sustained activity and also again after rest [1, 4].

Diplopia can be demonstrated by having the patient look laterally for about 30 seconds, leading to evident eye muscle fatigue [3]. The lid ptosis can improve by applying cold on the affected eye ("ice pack test"). Also, passively lifting a ptotic lid may cause the opposite lid to fall ("enhanced ptosis") [1]. Cogan's lid twitch—a pathognomic sign in MG—is described as the brief twitch seen in an eyelid that is elevated after rest [4, 5].

A useful functional test for dysarthria implies asking the patient to speak aloud without interruption producing nasality and/or hoarseness [6].

To test the limb muscle weakness, the patient should be asked to maintain for 3 minutes a horizontally stretched position of arms, hands, and fingers. In patients with MG, this test will lead to shaking or a gradual drooping of arms, hands, or fingers. Also, patients should be able to do knee bends or rise from a chair repeatedly without any support, 20 times.

Importantly, vital capacity and peak flow measurements should be assessed in all myasthenic patients [6].

4. Clinical classification

Several scoring systems of myasthenic signs or the global state of the patient have been proposed including the Osserman classification, myasthenia gravis composite (MGC) scale, and quantitative myasthenia gravis (QMG) score [6]. However, currently the most widely accepted is the MG Foundation of America (MGFA) Clinical Classification which divides MG into five main classes and several subclasses [3, 5] as follows:

- **Class I**: Any ocular muscle weakness; may have weakness of eye closure. All other muscle strength is normal.

- **Class II**: Mild weakness affecting muscles other than ocular muscles; may also have ocular muscle weakness of any severity.
    - **IIa**. Predominantly affecting the limb, axial muscles, or both. May also have lesser involvement of oropharyngeal muscles.
    - **IIb**. Predominantly affecting the oropharyngeal, respiratory muscles, or both. May also have lesser or equal involvement of the limb, axial muscles, or both.
- **Class III**: Moderate weakness affecting muscles other than ocular muscles; may also have ocular muscle weakness of any severity.
    - **IIIa**. Predominantly affecting the limb, axial muscles, or both. May also have lesser involvement of oropharyngeal muscles.
    - **IIIb**. Predominantly affecting the oropharyngeal and respiratory muscles or both. May also have lesser or equal involvement of the limb, axial muscles, or both.
- **Class IV**: Severe weakness affecting muscles other than ocular muscles; may also have ocular muscle weakness of any severity.
    - **IVa**. Predominantly affecting the limb, axial muscles, or both. May also have lesser involvement of oropharyngeal muscles.
    - **IVb**. Predominantly affecting oropharyngeal, respiratory muscles, or both. May also have lesser or equal involvement of limb, axial muscles, or both.
- **Class V**: Defined as a state requiring intubation, with or without mechanical ventilation, except when employed during routine postoperative management. The use of a feeding tube without intubation places the patient in Class IVb [14].

5. Myasthenia gravis subtypes and specific clinical situations

Ocular MG (OMG). Myasthenic weakness that remains restricted to the ocular muscles for more than 2 years is defined as OMG [15] (**Figure 1**). Although most patients with OMG also present concomitant weakness of the orbicularis oculi muscles, this is not considered as evidence of generalization [5]. Remission may be seen in about 20% of these patients; however, it has to be noted that recurrences are possible even after 20 years [4, 5].

Generalized MG (GMG) can be further subclassified in early-onset (EOMG) and late-onset (LOMG) disease, with the cutoff age usually set at age 40. EOMG patients are more often women, typically presenting anti-AChR antibodies and thymus hyperplasia, while LOMG patients are more frequently male and have MuSK antibodies in addition to anti-AChR antibodies [1].

MuSK-antibody myasthenia gravis (MuSK-MG). MuSK antibodies have been reported in up to 50% of seronegative autoimmune MG cases [16] as well as in OMG [17]. MuSK-MG occurs predominately in women from adolescence through middle age [1, 5]. The anti-MuSK phenotype has a distinct clinical syndrome with prominent weakness in the cranial, bulbar, and respiratory muscles, frequently with moderate to severe atrophy of these clinically affected muscles (especially facial and genioglossus muscles) [1, 4, 5, 18]. Thus, the major complaints of these patients

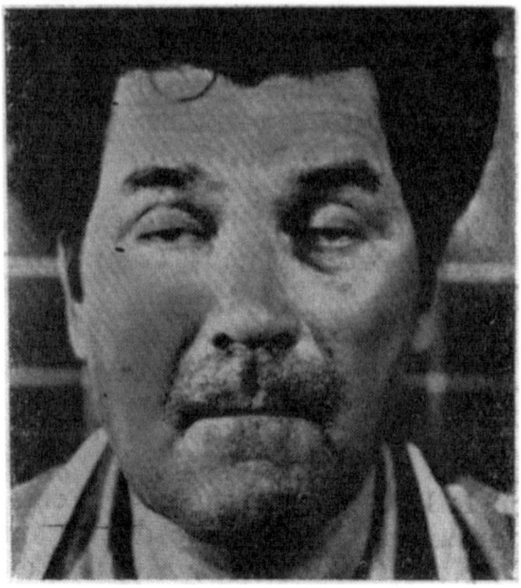

Figure 1.
Ocular myasthenia gravis.

include dyspnea, nasal speech, and dysphagia leading sometimes to an important weight loss [2]. Some patients also present weakness of the neck extensor. Typically, there is little to no ocular muscle weakness and only a mild involvement of the limb muscles. It is important to mention that, in these patients, the myasthenic symptoms are more severe than in non-MuSK-MG individuals, with more frequent respiratory crises [5]. In MuSK-MG thymic pathology is mostly absent or minimal [19].

Seronegative MG is defined by the absence of both anti-AChR and anti-MuSK antibodies ("double-seronegative MG"). These cases are clinically heterogeneous, but their frequency is particularly low. It has to be noted that some of these patients may have low-affinity anti-AChR antibodies that can only be detected using specialized assays [1].

Thymoma-associated MG. Thymic pathology (thymic lymphofollicular hyperplasia and thymoma) occurs in 80–90% of MG patients and is typically milder in seronegative MG [20]. It was reported that over 10% of patients with MG have a thymoma and, conversely, that 35% of thymoma patients have MG [5]. Thymoma-associated MG, also termed paraneoplastic MG, is a seropositive MG subtype which occurs primarily after the third life decade and is equally frequent in males and females. Patients with this MG subtype have a more severe disease with lower rates of remission and higher mortality (30%) than patients without thymoma [1, 5, 6].

Transient neonatal myasthenia gravis (**TNMG**) occurs in approximately 15% of infants born to mothers with autoimmune MG, as the anti-AChR antibodies get transferred across the placenta. The most common symptoms are feeble cry, ptosis, facial weakness, difficulty in feeding, respiratory weakness, and, in some cases, cyanosis. Rarely, affected infants present arthrogryposis (joint contracture) causing prolonged immobility in utero. It was found that the symptom severity in the newborn is not related to the severity of symptoms in the mother. These myasthenic manifestations resolve within the first month of life with acetylcholine esterase inhibitors [1, 5].

Juvenile myasthenia gravis (JMG) is defined as the onset of immune-mediated MG before age 18 [21] (**Figure 2**). These patients represent about 15% of the

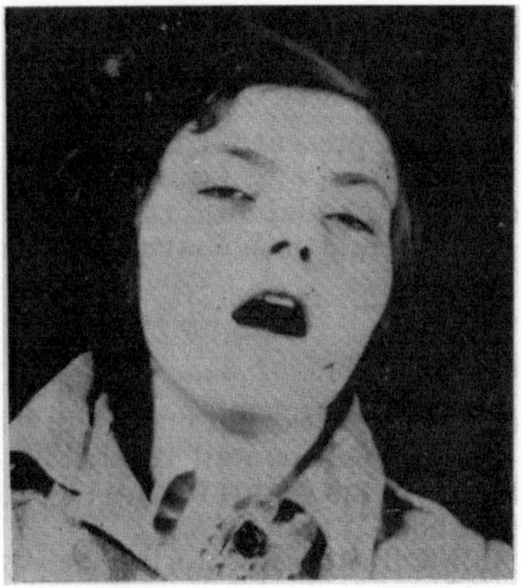

Figure 2.
Myasthenic crisis in juvenile myasthenia gravis.

autoimmune MG cases, being particularly uncommon in the first year of life. JMG is rarely associated with thymomas and has a high rate of spontaneous remission [1].

Congenital myasthenic syndromes (CMS) are caused by genetic (mostly autosomal recessive) abnormalities of the NMT, leading to fluctuating or persistent hypotonia of the ocular, bulbar, or limb muscles; in infancy it may cause arthrogryposis, delayed motor milestones, and unexplained apnea episodes. The weakness usually worsens during adolescence but then often stabilizes; however, prominent myopathy and scoliosis may be present [1, 4].

Lambert-Eaton myasthenic syndrome (LEMS). LEMS is a rare autoimmune disorder resulting from impaired release of ACh by the presynaptic terminal of the NM junction and in the autonomic ganglia. By definition, LEMS is associated with the presence of anti-presynaptic P/Q type voltage-gated calcium channels (VGCC) antibodies. Clinically, LEMS has an insidious onset - usually characterized by muscle tenderness - followed by progressive development of weakness and fatigue [1, 4, 5]. The most frequent symptoms found in LEMS include abnormal fatigue, weakness of the proximal muscles (particularly in the legs), hyporeflexia, and, dysautonomic manifestations (dry mouth, orthostatic hypotension constipation, and impotence). Some patients may present facilitation of strength after brief, isometric contraction and decline of strength after sustained activity. LEMS is classically associated with underlying malignancy or autoimmune disease. It was reported that in about 75% of men and 30% of women, this is a paraneoplastic condition accompanying in most of the cases (80%) a small cell lung cancer. The disease can also occur with other malignancies such as lymphoproliferative disorders, malignant thymoma, and rarely carcinoma of the breast, stomach, colon, prostate, and bladder [4, 5].

Pregnancy. MG may improve, worsen, or remain stable during pregnancy; however, a significant risk of deterioration in the puerperium was reported [1, 4]. Severe respiratory insufficiency can be triggered by the physical stress of labor and delivery; similarly, patients with eclampsia during pregnancy have a higher risk of complications of both conditions, considering, for example, that magnesium sulfate cannot be used in MG patients [5]. It should also be noted that a newborn from a myasthenic pregnancy has a higher risk to develop TNMG (see above). Currently, women with MG are advised to delay pregnancy until after the disease is stable [1, 4] (**Table 2**).

Myasthenia gravis subtypes and specific clinical situations	Notes
Ocular MG	• Weakness restricted to the ocular muscles
Generalized MG	• Subclassified in early-onset and late-onset MG • Typically associated with anti-AChR antibodies
MuSK-antibody myasthenia gravis	• Prominent weakness in the cranial, bulbar, and respiratory muscles • Myasthenic symptoms more severe than in non-MuSK-MG patients
Seronegative MG	• Rare • Clinically heterogeneous
Thymoma-associated MG	• 80–90% of MG patients also present thymic pathology • Lower rates of remission and higher mortality
Transient neonatal myasthenia gravis	• May occur in infants born to mothers with autoimmune MG • The myasthenic symptoms resolve within the first month of life with treatment
Juvenile myasthenia gravis	• The disease onset occurs before age 18 • High rate of spontaneous remission
Congenital myasthenic syndromes	• Caused by genetic (mostly autosomal recessive) abnormalities of the NMT
Lambert-Eaton myasthenic syndrome	• Associated with anti-presynaptic P/Q type VGCC antibodies • Frequent symptoms: fatigue, weakness of the proximal muscles (particularly in the legs), hyporeflexia, and dysautonomic manifestations • Associated with underlying malignancy or other autoimmune disease
Pregnancy	• MG may improve, worsen, or remain stable during pregnancy • Women with MG are advised to delay pregnancy until after the disease is stable

Table 2.
Myasthenia gravis subtypes and specific clinical situations—Summarized features.

Author details

Jianu Catalin[1,2]*, Jianu Silviana[3] and Barsan Claudia[2]

1 Department of Neurology, "Victor Babes" University of Medicine and Pharmacy, Timisoara, Romania

2 Department of Neurology, Clinical Emergency County Hospital, Timisoara, Romania

3 Department of Ophthalmology, Military Emergency Hospital, Timisoara, Romania

*Address all correspondence to: dcjianu@yahoo.com

References

[1] Daroff RB, Jankovic J, Mazziotta JC, Scott L, editors. Bradley's Neurology in Clinical Practice. London, New York, Oxford, Philadephia, St. Louis, Sydney, Toronto: Elsevier; 2016. ISBN: 978-0-323-28783-8. Pomeroy Seventh Edition

[2] Angelini C, Martignago S, Biscigli M, Albertini E. Myasthenia gravis with anti-MuSK antibodies: Clinical features and histopathological changes. In: Pruitt JA, editor. A Look into Myasthenia Gravis. Rijeka: InTech; 2011. ISBN 978-953-307-821-2

[3] Trouth AJ, Dabi A, Solieman N, Kurukumbi M, Kalyanam J. Myasthenia gravis: A review. Autoimmune Disease. 2012;**2012**:874680

[4] Clarke C, Howard R, Rossor M, Shorvon S, editors. Neurology: A Queen Square Textbook. Oxford: Blackwell Publishing Ltd.; 2009. ISBN: 978-1-405-13443-9

[5] Engel AG, editor. Myasthenia Gravis and Myasthenic Disorders. Oxford: Oxford University Press; 2012. ISBN-13: 9780199738670

[6] Kaminski HJ. Myasthenia Gravis and Related Disorders. Totowa, New Jersey: Humana Press Inc; 2003. ISBN 1-58829-058-1

[7] Scherer K, Bedlack RS, Simel DL. Does this patient have myasthenia gravis? JAMA. 2005;**293**(15):1906-1914

[8] Grob D, Brunner N, Namba T, Pagala M. Lifetime course of myasthenia gravis. Muscle & Nerve. 2008;**37**(2):141-149

[9] Beekman R, Kuks JBM, Oosterhuis HJGH. Myasthenia gravis: Diagnosis and follow-up of 100 consecutive patients. Journal of the Neurological Sciences. 1997;**244**:112-118

[10] Myasthenia Gravis Foundation of America. Myasthenia Gravis: A Manual for the Health Care Provider. 2008. Available from: http://www.myasthenia.org/docs/MGFA_ProfessionalManual.pdf

[11] Grob D. Course and management of myasthenia gravis. JAMA. 1953;**153**:529-532

[12] Koopman WJ, Wiebe S, Colton-Hudson A, Moosa T, Smith D, Bach D, et al. Prediction of aspiration in myasthenia gravis. Muscle & Nerve. 2004;**29**(2):256-260

[13] Romi F, Skeie GO, Gilhus NE. Striational antibodies in myasthenia gravis: Reactivity and possible clinical significance. Archives of Neurology. 2005;**62**(3):442-446

[14] Jaretzki A 3rd, Barohn RJ, Ernstoff RM, Kaminski HJ, Keesey JC, Penn AS, et al. Myasthenia gravis: Recommendations for clinical research standards. Task Force of the Medical Scientific Advisory Board of the Myasthenia Gravis Foundation of America. The Annals of Thoracic Surgery. 2000;**70**(1):327-334

[15] Kupersmith MJ, Latkany R, Homel P. Development of generalized disease at 2 years in patients with ocular myasthenia gravis. Archives of Neurology. 2003;**60**:243-248

[16] Guptill JT, Sanders DB. Update on muscle-specific tyrosine kinase antibody positive myasthenia gravis. Current Opinion in Neurology. 2010;**23**(5):530-535

[17] Bau V, Hanisch F, Hain B, Zierz S. Ocular involvement in MuSK antibody-positive myasthenia gravis. Klinische Monatsblätter für Augenheilkunde. 2006;**223**:81-83

[18] Evoli A, Tonali PA, Padua L, Monaco ML, Scuderi F, Batocchi AP, et al. Clinical correlates with anti-MuSK antibodies in generalized seronegative myasthenia gravis. Brain. 2003;**126** (Pt 10):2304-2311

[19] Lauriola L, Ranelletti F, Maggiano N, Guerriero M, Punzi C, Marsili F, et al. Thymus changes in anti-MuSK-positive and -negative myasthenia gravis. Neurology. 2005;**64**(3):536-538

[20] Willcox N, Schluep M, Ritter MA, Newsom-Davis J. The thymus in seronegative myasthenia gravis patients. Journal of Neurology. 1991;**238**:256-261

[21] Andrews PI, Sanders DB. Juvenile myasthenia gravis. In: Jones HR, DeVivo DC, Darras BT, editors. Neuromuscular Disorders of Infancy, Childhood, and Adolescence. Boston: Butterworth Heinemann; 2002. pp. 575-597. ISBN-13: 978-0750671903

Chapter 9

The Effect of Atmospheric Pollution on the Thymus

Martha Ustarroz-Cano, Marisol López-Ángel, Nelly López-Valdez, Isabel García-Peláez and Teresa I. Fortoul

Abstract

Air pollution is a high-risk factor in megacities' dwellers because of its effects on health. One of the most important components of the pollution is particulate matter (PM) on which metals are adhered. One element adhered to its surfaces is vanadium (V), and through this route, PM reaches the respiratory system, then the systemic circulation and the rest of the organs. Vanadium is released in the atmosphere as a consequence of the combustion of fossil fuels. Vanadium pentoxide is the compound liberated after the combustion and adhered into PM. Previous studies from our group have reported effects on diverse systems in a mouse model. Besides the morphological changes in the spleen and the decreased function of the immune humoral response, the thymus was also affected. Vanadium inhalation diminished thymic dendritic cells (DCs) and the biomarkers: CD11c and MHCII; in addition, thymic cytoarchitecture changed, demonstrated by cytokeratin-5, and also, modification in the expression of 3-nitrotyrosine was observed. Our findings suggest that autoreactive T cells could be released into the systemic circulation and favor the increase in autoimmune diseases in cities with high concentrations of PM.

Keywords: thymus, vanadium inhalation, dendritic cells, oxidative stress, nitrosative stress, autoreactive T cells

1. Introduction

The air is the source of a variety of pollutants such as gases and particulate matter (PM). Particulate matter sources are construction sites, unpaved roads, forest fires, volcanic eruptions, power plants and a variety of combustion processes. Internal combustion motors are an important source of PM, especially those with old technology and without the proper maintenance [1]. The PM size is linked to their capacity to produce health problems since the smallest can reach the deepest lung spaces, the alveoli, and translocate into the blood stream. Doing so, PM reaches diverse systems and organs producing physiological modifications. One of the systems affected by PM is the lymphoid. Few papers report the direct effect of the PM in the Thymus, which is a central actor in the future definition of the immune response and self-recognition and self-tolerance, increasing the risk for developing allergic or autoimmune diseases [2–6].

Dendritic cells play an important function as mediators between innate and adaptive responses and they are susceptible to the effect of some of the components of the PM, such as transition metals, especially vanadium (V) which is liberated into the atmosphere by the combustion of fossil fuels [7]. One of the mechanisms by which V produces its effects is by oxidative or nitrosative stress and this mechanism is also proposed as the way by which the immune system is affected. In this report we describe the effect of vanadium, as a component of PM, and its oxidative and nitrosative effect on the structure and cells of the thymus.

2. Oxidative and nitrosative stress

Reactive oxygen and nitrogen species (RONS) are produced by cells normally as a result of their metabolism, and they function as key molecules in the maintenance of homeostasis by participating in various signaling pathways [8].

ROS include non-radical molecules derived from the molecular reduction of oxygen such as hydrogen peroxide (H_2O_2) and hypochlorous acid (HOCl) and oxygen-derived free radicals, such as: superoxide anion ($^{\cdot}O_2$) and hydroxyl radical ($^{\cdot}OH$) among others. The RNS include non-radical molecules such as nitrous acid (HNO_2), peroxynitrite (ONOO-) and free radicals derived from nitrogen such as nitric oxide ($^{\cdot}NO$) and nitrogen dioxide ($^{\cdot}NO_2$) among others [9, 10].

It is important to note that free radicals can be derived from many elements and molecules in addition to oxygen and nitrogen, such as hydrogen, carbon and transition metals such as iron and copper. RONS are important from the biological point of view due to their reactivity, which allows them to interact with different biomolecules [11, 12].

In the cells, reactive oxygen species are produced mainly through mitochondrial respiration, although there are other sources such as NADPH oxidases, microsomes, peroxisomes and other enzymes of metabolism such as CYP450 [11–13]. Reactive nitrogen species, such as $^{\cdot}NO$, are produced from the metabolism of L-arginine in a process catalyzed by nitric acid synthases (NOS). By combining the radical $^{\cdot}NO$ with $^{\cdot}O_2$, the anion peroxynitrite, which is reactive nitrogen species, can be formed [11]. The latter reveals the close relationship between the production of ROS and RNS.

Cells have physiological mechanisms that usually counteract the presence of reactive species by keeping them at low levels: antioxidants. These maintain the RONS levels below the toxic threshold. Under conditions in which the antioxidants are in imbalance with RONS, and the balance is tilted in favor of the latter, oxidative/nitrosative stress occurs [12, 14, 15].

As mentioned above, all species are able to interact with biomolecules (nucleic acids, proteins, lipids and carbohydrates), and under conditions of oxidative or nitrosative stress, RONS produce negative effects on them, altering their biological functions. Lipid peroxidation, protein modification and DNA oxidation are clear examples of the damage produced by the interaction with RONS [16].

External factors have been identified, such as the exposure to pollution, which may induce an increase in the production of RONS, causing oxidative and nitrosative stress [17]. Within the multiple components of the pollution, suspended particles and the metals, attached to them, increase the production of both types of species in the cells inducing oxidative and/or nitrosative stress. This stress has been associated with adverse effects such as inflammation, cytotoxicity and cellular damage in general [18]. It has been identified that soluble metals that are part of the particles such as iron (Fe), nickel (Ni), cobalt (Co), copper (Cu), chromium (Cr) and vanadium (V) generate these effects [19, 20].

What are the mechanisms involved in the formation of RONS by the participation of metals? The metals can induce the formation of free radicals through the Fenton reaction, in which the metal reacts with hydrogen peroxide (H_2O_2)

producing the hydroxyl radical ($^{\cdot}OH$) and an ion of the oxidized metal. It has been identified that metals such as cobalt (Co), chromium (Cr), nickel (Ni), iron (Fe) and vanadium (V) can be part of this reaction. Another mechanism by which metals produce free radicals is the Haber-Weiss reaction; in it an oxidized metal ion is reduced by superoxide ($^{\cdot}O_2$) and subsequently reacts with H_2O_2 producing hydroxyl radical. Metals such as cobalt, chromium and vanadium can participate in this reaction [21, 22].

The study of oxidizing and nitrosative stress is relevant due to the consequences that may have on biomolecules, and at a higher level, on the functions of organisms; this study can be approached with different methods.

One of the most used tools is the detection of products modified by reactive species, since they are more stable than the species themselves. Among the products that can be detected are those of oxidized lipids (such as aldehydes and ketones), proteins (as carbonylated and nitrosylated amino acid residues) and nucleic acids (such as 8-oxo-2-deoxyguanosine). An important utility of the ROS and RNS markers is their potential to identify the nature of the oxidant itself [9].

3-Nitrotyrosine (3-NT) has been identified as one of the most relevant markers, which shows the modification in proteins as a consequence of nitrosative stress. This marker is formed as a product of the nitration of tyrosine residues in proteins and occurs through the action of a nitrosative agent (ONOO-, $^{\cdot}NO$, HNO_2, etc.) that is added to the amino group (NO_2) of the polypeptide chain, leading to the nitration of tyrosine residues. This marker can be identified by immunoassays such as immunohistochemistry, immunofluorescence, ELISA [23].

It has been reported that 3-nitrotyrosine is involved in different pathological conditions such as inflammation, endothelial dysfunction, cardiovascular, liver, neurodegenerative, immunological diseases, aging, among others [23, 24].

3. Thymus and vanadium

The thymus is a capsulated primary lymphoid organ to which immature peripheral T-lymphocytes, from the bone marrow, arrives to complete its maturation and immune capacitation. It is located in the mediastinum; it has two lobules that originate from the third and fourth branchial poaches. In humans the thymus is fully formed and functional at birth and it reduces its size after puberty; however, it remains functional.

Histologically, it has a connective tissue capsule that extends into the parenchyma dividing it in incomplete lobules. In each lobule medulla and cortex are well delimited. The cortex is highly basophilic when the thymus is stained with hematoxylin and eosin as a consequence of the numerous and rapidly dividing immature T-lymphocytes called thymocytes, while the medulla is less basophilic because the thymocytes density decreases. Other cells in the thymus structure are the epithelial cells, located in the cortex-cortical epithelial thymic cells (cTEC)-, the medullary epithelial thymic cells (mTEC)-in the medulla-, also dendritic cells (DCs) located in the corticomedullary zone and in the medulla in addition of widely distributed macrophages. Small spherical-shaped structures, formed by mTEC, identified as Hassall's corpuscles -are thymic unique structures; its function is to regulate the production and maturation of the regulatory-T cells (Tregs). The thymus has a hematothymic barrier constituted by the vascular face of the endothelial cells from the cortex continuous capillaries, the basal lamina from the cortex continuous capillaries and the cTEC. Its function is to prevent the contact of the circulating antigens with the cortical thymocytes [25].

3.1 Positive and negative thymus selection

The maturation process from thymocytes to immunocompetent T cells depends on the cortical and medullar thymic microenvironments that is established by the cTEC, mTEC, and DC. The cTEC positively select the T-lymphocytes that recognize the major histocompatibility complex (MHC), so the selected T-lymphocytes are CD4+ or CD8+. The mTEC and the DCs are involved in negative T-cell selection and in establishing self-tolerance by eliminating through apoptosis, the lymphocytes which strongly recognize self-antigens, preventing autoreactive clones. Both processes area highly ordinated and rely on the sequential and quantitative expression of markers such as CD4, CD8, T-cell receptors (TCR1, TCR2) as well as of changes in the glycosylation of the membrane proteins on the lymphocytes in the process of maturation [26, 27].

3.2 Dendritic cells

Dendritic cells (DCs) are antigen -presenting cells (APCs) from the bone marrow. They are a heterogeneous population of cells which are identify because their surfaces biomarkers, cytokines production and location. Their progenitors could be myeloid or lymphoid. DCs are recognized by its typical dendritic morphology and by the expression of CD11c. As all of the other APCs, MHCII is expressed on its surface [28]. The differentiation and function of the DCs could be modulated by different growth factors and cytokines. There are three types: cDCs, the conventional type; pDCs, the plasmacytoid type; and mDCs, the monocyte-derived cells [29].

DCs are a bridge between innate and adaptive immune response. When they are immature its location is the skin and peripheral tissues and when an antigen is captured the cells migrate to present the antigen to the T cells. The thymus DCs and the mTEC are responsible of the thymocytes negative selection; in the medullae the single T cells (SP) interact with the DCs and with the mTEC that present them self-antigens with and immunogenic potential. The T-cell receptor (TCR) from the SP thymocytes recognizes the cells with MHC restriction and high affinity to self-antigens to eliminate them by apoptosis. This is the main mechanism to eliminate autoreactive clones and to establish central tolerance [29].

As it was previous mentioned V could damage health. Previous reports from our group demonstrated that, -in experimental model- mice that inhale V have damages in different systems including the immune system which induces changes in the cortex-medullae ratio [30, 31]. Other observed effect was in the spleen and in the humoral response [32].

Because of the morphological changes in the thymus as a consequence of the V-exposure, we decided to explore the changes in the expression of CD11c and MHCII on the DCs distribution.

We have developed a CD-1 mouse inhalation experimental model to assess systemic effects of PM. We used CD-1 mice (8-weeks-old, 33 + 2 g) from the vivarium of the School of medicine. The animals were randomly placed in acrylic chambers connected to an ultra-nebulizer (UltraNeb99 Devilbiss, Somerset, Philadelphia, USA), the exposure schedule consisted of V_2O_5 0.02 M (Sigma, St. Louis, Missouri, USA) in saline, 1 hour twice a week for 4 weeks. The ultra-nebulizer with the size of the particle emitted being less than 5 μm (range 0.5–5 μm) at a flow rate of 10 L/min. The concentration in the chamber was 1436 $\mu m/m^3$ [30, 31]. Mice were sacrificed at the end of each exposure week, the thymus was extracted and CD11c was detected by conventional immunohistochemistry. Other thymuses were processed for cytometry for CD11c+ and MHCII+. To obtain the enough cells the Baba method was modified [33]. Briefly, mice were sacrificed, thymus were extracted, macerated and submitted to enzymic digestion to obtain a homogenate, by magnetic cell sorting (MACS) the CD11c+ and MHCII+, cells were separated. The cells from the 3rd week of exposure were selected for cytometry because previous result indicated that in this period of time thymus changes were more evident.

The observed changes in CD11c are shown in **Figure 1**. In controls more CD11c+ cells were noticed compared with the exposed mice. The findings were supported with the densitometric results (GraphPad Prism Software, V5, 2007, La Jolla, CA) that showed a diminished presence of the CD11c+ in the medullae as the time of the exposure progress.

Flow cytometry showed that levels of CD11c+ and MHCII+ were significantly decreased in the V-exposed mice as compared with controls. The loss was both in terms of number and in mean fluorescence intensity (MIF) values. In brief, V-inhalation decreased the thymic CD11C+ and MHCII+ cells as the exposure time increased [4]. An explanation for our findings could be the V-oxidative capacity which has been previously reported by our group and by other authors [34, 35]. Oxidative stress could affect the liberation of pro-inflammatory transcription factors by the CD11c cells. The thymus dysfunction could by in the negative selection of the T cells that, in turn, could alter the interaction of CD4 lymphocytes with the MHCII protein on the DCs. Such changes could then promote the development of autoimmune responses as suggested by Chang and indirectly by Zouali [36, 37], who hypothesized that an epigenetic effect from urban air pollutants led to altered immune cell phenotypes that, in turn, favors the development of autoimmunity. Further studies are planned to investigate this topic.

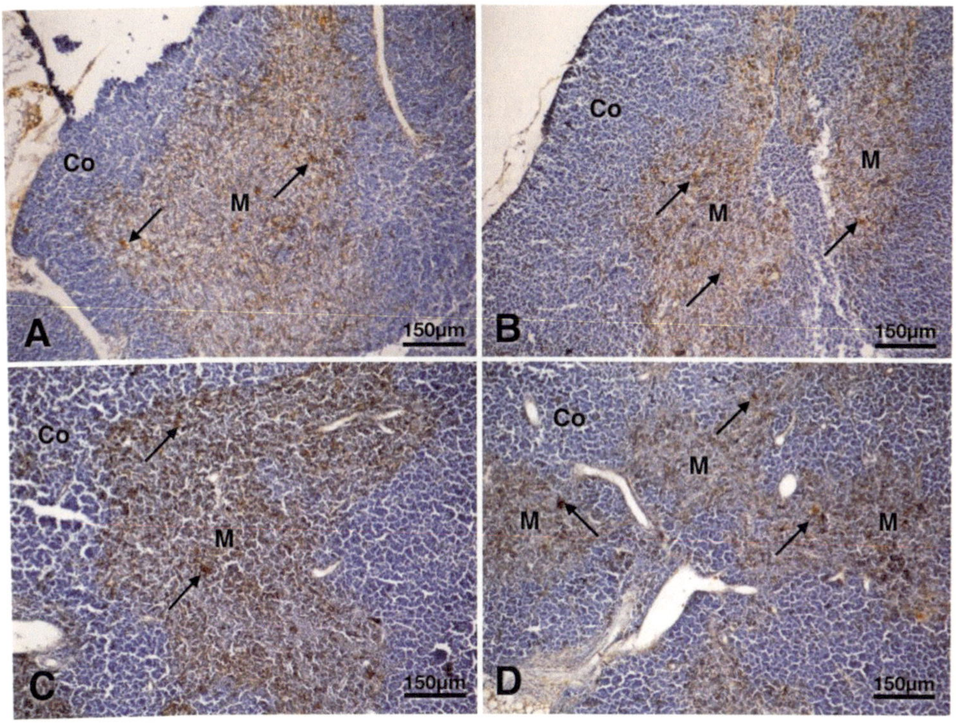

Figure 1.
CD11c expression in thymus. In control and V-exposed mice, ocher color stained (arrows) cells CD11c+ were distributed mainly in the medulla (M); scanty positive cells were present in the cortex (Co). Representative photomicrographs from (A, C) control (B, D) 4-week-V-exposed. (A, C) Reveal a higher presence of CD11c+ cells compared to the shown in (B, D).

3.3 Thymic epithelial cells

Previous studies have demonstrated the interdependence of TEC and the thymocytes to maintain the thymic microenvironment integrity. TEC are APCs distributed in the cortex (cTEC) and in the medullae (mTEC). cTEC select the thymocytes that express TCR and recognize self-MHC. The remaining cells are eliminated by apoptosis; this positive selection takes place in the cortex. mTEC with DCs are in charge of the negative selection of T cells and to establish central tolerance, as well as helping to regulate the production of regulatory T cells (Treg) [26, 27]. Previous studies from our group have demonstrated that V exposure change the thymic

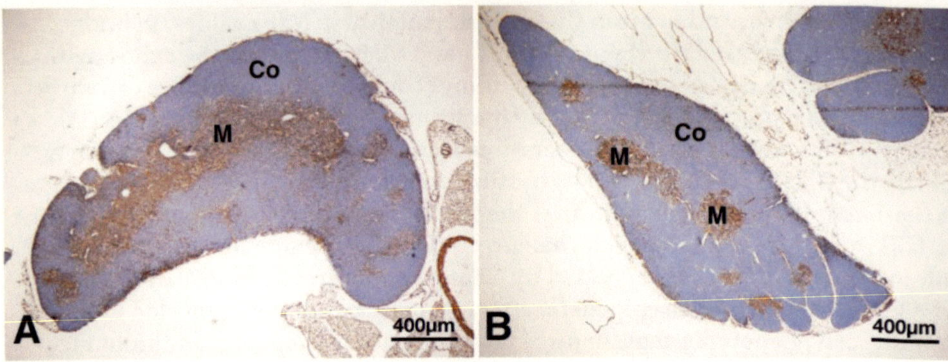

Figure 2.
K5 expression in the thymus. Representative photomicrographs from: (A) control and (B) 2-week-V-exposed. Positive K5 cells are located in the medullae (M) and some in the cortex (Co), B. K5+ cells located in the medulla (M) but also in the cortex (Co).

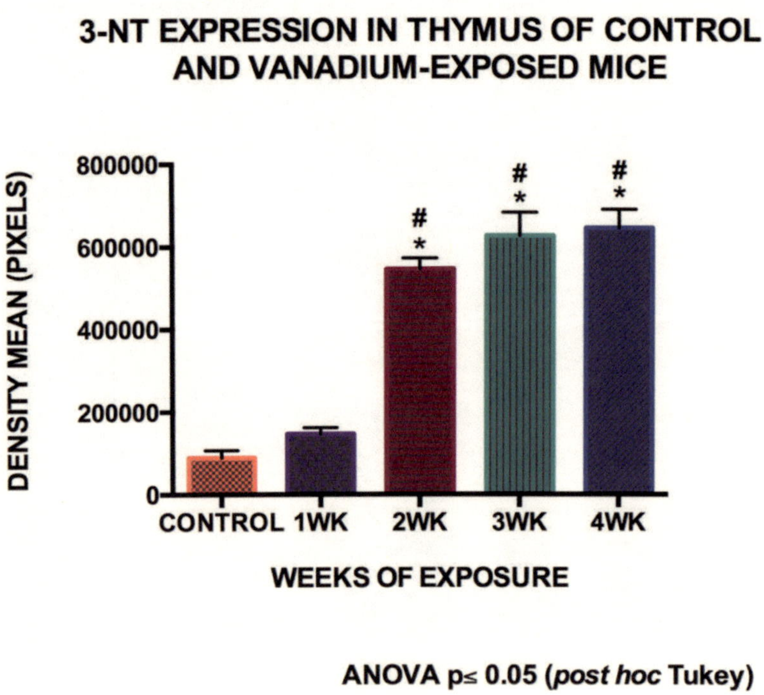

Figure 3.
Density means of 3-NT cells in the thymus (density mean ± SEM of pixels/mm^2). Density values increased in V-exposed mice from week 1 to week 4. ANOVA (Tukey's) $p \leq 0.05$.

cortex/medullae ratio and by using cytokeratin-5 (K5) as a marker, the mistaken location of the K5+ cells in the medulla was demonstrated **Figure 2** [4, 30].

The density mean showed the changes in the presence of K5+, ocher-stain cells that increased during the first week of exposure compared with controls; however, the stain density at weeks 2 and 4 had a slight decrease but never reached the control values $p < 0.05$. These results showed that V produced changes in thymus cytoarchitecture, in addition of an increase in K5+ cells, changes that suggest that the T-cell selection was disrupted by V-inhalation [5]. Also, the presence of nitrosative stress as possible explanation of our findings was explored with 3-nitrotyrosine (3-NT) [38].

Our unpublished data demonstrated an increase time-dependent in the whole thymus tissue of 3-NT (**Figure 3**).

4. Conclusions

Air pollution affects the thymus. V inhalation induces nitrosative stress a decrease in DCs, the expression of CD11c and MHCII and mTEC increase, which could implicate that the negative and the positive selection were not properly completed. All these changes could allow that autoreactive clones were liberated to the blood stream and the incidence in autoimmune diseases rises in the dwellers of polluted cities [39].

Author details

Martha Ustarroz-Cano, Marisol López-Ángel, Nelly López-Valdez,
Isabel García-Peláez and Teresa I. Fortoul*
Department of Cellular and Tissular Biology, School of Medicine, National Autonomous University of Mexico (UNAM), Mexico City, México

*Address all correspondence to: fortoul@unam.mx

References

[1] Riveros HG, Cabrera E, Ovalle P. Vehicle inspection and maintenance, and air pollution in Mexico City. Transportation Research Part D. 2001;7:73-80. DOI: 10.1016/S1361-9209(01)00010-4

[2] Bleck B, Tse DB, Gordon T, Ahsan MR, Reibman J. Diesel exhaust particulate-treated human bronchial epithelial cells up-regulate Jagged-1 and OX40 ligand in myeloid dendritic cells vía thymus stromal lymphopoietin. Journal of Immunology. 2010;**185**:6636-6645. DOI: 10.4049/jimmunol.1000719

[3] Yan L, Gong C, Ying L, Fu W, Liu S, Dai J, et al. PM 2.5 affects establishment of immune tolerance in newborn mice by reducing PD-L1 expression. Journal of Biosciences. 2019;**44**(2):1-8. DOI: 10.1007/s12038-019-9858-6

[4] Ustarroz-Cano M, Garcia-Pelaez I, Piñon-Zarate G, Herrera-Enriquez M, Soldevila G, Fortoul TI. CD11c decrease in mouse thymic dendritic cells after vanadium inhalation. Journal of Immunotoxicology. 2012;**9**:374-380. DOI: 10.3109/1547691X.2012.673181

[5] Ustarroz-Cano M, Garcia-Pelaez I, Cervates-Yepez S, Lopez-Valdez N, Fortoul TI. Thymic cytoarchitecture changes in mice exposed to vanadium. Journal of Immunotoxicology. 2017;**14**:9-14. DOI: 10.1080/1547691X.2016.1250848

[6] Gawda A, Majka G, Nowak B, Marcinkiewicz J. Air pollution, oxidative stress, and exacerbation of autoimmune diseases. Central European Journal of Immunology. 2017;**42**(3):3005-3012. DOI: 10.5114/ceji.2017.70975

[7] Fortoul TI, Rojas-Lemus M, Rodriguez-Lara V, Gonzalez-Villava A, Ustarroz-Cano M, Cano-Gutiérrez G, et al. Overview of environmental and occupational vanadium exposure and associated health outcomes: An article based on a presentation at the 8th international symposium of vanadium chemistry. Biological chemistry and toxicology, Washington DC, August 15-18, 2012. Journal of Immunotoxicology. 2014;**11**(1):13-18. DOI: 10.3109/1547691X.2013.789940

[8] Manke A, Wang L, Rojanasakul Y. Mechanisms of nanoparticle-induced oxidative stress and toxicity. BioMed Research International. 2013;**2013**:1-15. DOI: 10.1155/2013/942916

[9] Dalle-Donne I, Scaloni A, Giustarini D, Cavarra E, Tell G, Lungarella G, et al. Proteins as biomarkers of oxidative/nitrosative stress in diseases: The contribution of redox proteomics. Mass Spectrometry Reviews. 2005;**24**:55-99. DOI: 10.1002/mas.20006

[10] Di Meo S, Reed TT, Venditti P, Victor VM. Role of ROS and RNS sources in physiological and pathological conditions. Oxidative Medicine and Cellular Longevity. 2016;**2016**:1-44. DOI: 10.1155/2016/1245049

[11] Cárdenas-Rodríguez N, Pedraza-Chaverri J. Especies reactivas de oxígeno y sistemas antioxidantes: Aspectos básicos. Educación química. 2006;**17**(2):164-173

[12] Birben E, Sahiner UM, Sackesen C, Erzurum S, Kalayci O. Oxidative stress and antioxidant defense. World Allergy Organization Journal. 2012;**5**(1):9-19. DOI: 10.1097/WOX.0b013e3182439613

[13] Cutler RG, Plummer J, Chowdhury K, Heward C. Oxidative stress profiling. Part II. Theory, technology, and practice. Annals of the New York Academy of Sciences. 2005;**1055**:136-158. DOI: 10.1196/annals.1323.031

[14] Kohen R, Nyska A. Oxidation of biological systems: Oxidative

stress phenomena, antioxidants, redox reactions, and methods for their quantification. Toxicologic Pathology. 2002;**30**(6):620-650. DOI: 10.1080/01926230290166724

[15] Ray PD, Huang BW, Tsuji Y. Reactive oxygen species (ROS) homeostasis and redox regulation in cellular signaling. Cellular Signaling. 2012;**24**(5):981-990. DOI: 10.1016/j.cellsig.2012.01.008

[16] Weidinger A, Kozlov A. Biological activities of reactive oxygen and nitrogen species: Oxidative stress versus signal transduction. Biomolecules. 2015;**5**:472-484. DOI: 10.3390/biom5020472

[17] Maura L, Bigagli E. Oxidative stress and air pollution exposure. Journal of Toxicology. 2011:1-9. DOI: 10.1155/2011/487074

[18] Li N, Sioutas C, Cho A, Schmitz D, Misra C, Sempf J, et al. Ultrafine particulate pollutants induce oxidative stress and mitochondrial damage. Environmental Health Perspectives. 2003;**111**(4):455-460. DOI: 10.1289/ehp.6000

[19] Knaapen AM, Shi T, Borm PJA, Schins RPF. Soluble metals as well as the insoluble particle fraction are involved in cellular DNA damage induced by particulate matter. Molecular and Cellular Biochemistry. 2002;**234-235**:317-326. DOI: 10.1023/A:1015970023889

[20] Leonard S, Harris G, Shi X. Metal-induced oxidative stress and signal transduction. Free Radical Biology & Medicine. 2004;**37**(12):1921-1942

[21] Valko M, Morris H, Cronin MTD. Metals, toxicity and oxidative stress. Current Medicinal Chemistry. 2005;**12**:1161-1208

[22] Jomova K, Baros S, Valko M. Redox active metal-induced oxidative stress in biological systems. Transition Metal Chemistry. 2012;**37**(2):127-134. DOI: 10.1007/s11243-012-9583-6

[23] Ahsan H. 3-Nitrotyrosine: A biomarker of nitrogen free radical species modified proteins in systemic autoimmunogenic conditions. Human Immunology. 2013;**74**(10):1392-1399. DOI: 10.1016/j.humimm.2013.06.009

[24] Sies H, Berndt C, Jones DP. Oxidative stress. Annual Review of Biochemistry. 2017;**86**(1): 715-748. DOI: 10.1146/annurev-biochem-061516-045037

Castell A, Herrera M, Ustarroz M. Tejido y órganos linfoides. In: Fortoul T, editor. Histología y Biología Celular. 3rd ed. Mexico City: Mc Graw Hill; 2017. pp. 173-189. ISBN: 978-607-15-1408-0

[25] Mouri Y, Nishijima H, Kawano H, Hirota F, Sakaguchi N, Morimoto J, et al. NF-κB-inducing kinase in thymic stroma establishes central tolerance by, orchestrating crosstalk with not only thymocytes but also dendritic cells. The Journal of immunology. 2014;**193**:4356-4367. DOI: 10.4049/jimmunol.1400389

[26] Ucar O, Rattay K. Promiscuous gene expression in the thymus: A matter of epigenetics, miRNA, and more? Frontiers in Immunology. 2015;**6**:93. DOI: 10.3389/fimmu.2015.00093

[27] Wu L, Liu YJ. Development of dendritic-cell lineages. Immunity. 2007;**26**:741-750. DOI: 10.1016/j.immuni.2007.06.006

[28] Chavez-Sanchez FR, Rivera-Jimenez J, Bottasso Lazareschi O. Respuesta inmunológica innata. In: Pavon-Romero L, Jimenez-Martinez MC, Garces Alvarez ME, editors. Inmunología Molecular, Celular y Traslacional. Wolters: Kluwer; 2016. pp. 72-85. ISBN: 978-84-16004-86-7

[29] Fortoul TI, Rodriguez-Lara V, Gonzalez-Villalva A, Rojas-Lemus M, Cano-Gutierrez G, Ustarroz-Cano M, et al. Vanadium inhalation in a mouse model for the understanding of air-suspended particle systemic repercussion. Journal of Biomedicine & Biotechnology. 2011;**2011**:951043. DOI: 10.1155/2011/951043

[30] Fortoul TI, Rodriguez-Lara V, Gonzalez-Villalva A, Rojas-Lemus M, Cano-Gutierrez G, Ustarroz-Cano M, et al. Inhalation of vanadium pentoxide and its effects in a mouse model. Inorganica Chimica Acta. 2014;**420**:8-15. DOI: 10.1016/j.ica.2014.03.027

[31] Piñon-Zarate G, Rodriguez-Lara V, Rojas-Lemus M, Martinez-Pedraza M, Gonzalez-Villalva A, Mussali-Galante P, et al. Vanadium pentoxide inhalation provokes germinal center hyperplasia and suppressed humoral immune response. Journal Immunol toxicol. 2008;**5**:115-122. DOI: 10.1080/15476910802085749

[32] Baba T, Nakamoto Y, Mukaida N. Crucial contribution of thymic sirpα+ conventional dendritic cells to central tolerance against blood-borne antigens in a CCR-dependent manner. Journal of Immunology. 2009;**183**:3053-3063. DOI: 10.4049/jimmunol.0900438

[33] Gusik TJ, Korbut R, Adame-Gusik T. Nitric oxide and superoxide in inflammation and immune regulation. Journal of Physiology and Pharmacology. 2003;**54**:469-487

[34] Cano Gutierrez G, Acevedo-Nava S, Santamaria A, Altamirano-Lozano M, Cano-Rodriguez MC, Fortoul TI. Hepatic megalocytosis due to vanadium inhalation: Participation of oxidative stress. Toxicology and Industrial Health. 2012;**28**:353-360. DOI: 10.1177/0748233711412424

[35] Chang C. The immune effects of naturally occurring and synthetic nanoparticles. Journal of Autoimmunity. 2010;**34**:J234-J246. DOI: 10.1016/j.jaut.2009.11.009

[36] Zouali M. Epigenetics in lupus. Annals of the New York Academy of Sciences. 2011;**1217**:154-165. DOI: 10.1111/j.1749-6632.2010.05831.x

[37] Garcia GA, Clavijo D, Mejia OR, Casariego CA, Garcia-Cardona A, Hernandez-Vela S, et al. Biología, patobiología, bioclínica y farmacoterapeítica de la di-metil-arginina asimetrica (ADMA) en la especie humana. Universitas Médica. 2006;**47**:335-348

[38] Fortoul TI, Rojas-Lemus M. Vanadium as an air pollutant. In: Fortoul TI, Avila-Costa MR, editors. Vanadium: Its Impact on Health. New York: Nova Science Publishers; 2007. pp. 1-6. ISBN: 1-60021-609-9

Chapter 10

Essential Oils of *Thymbra capitata* and *Thymus hyemalis* and Their Uses Based on Their Bioactivity

Ana Belén Sabater-Jara, María Pina Funes, María Angeles Pedreño and Sarai Belchí-Navarro

Abstract

Essential oils (EO) are volatile compounds produced by the secondary metabolism of aromatic plants. They are complex mixtures whose main components are synthesized by the mevalonic acid and the methyl erythritol phosphate pathways, which lead to the biosynthesis of terpenes, and the shikimic acid pathway, responsible for the biosynthesis of phenylpropanoid compounds. In nature, EOs are stored in the aerial parts of the plant, being of vital importance for their survival due to their antimicrobial properties. In addition, EOs provide protection against herbivores to the aromatic plants and allow them to repel or attract insects because of their strong fragrance, as well as compete with other plants of the same environment. Humans have exploited the properties of their EOs since ancient times, being used as medicinal remedies, among other uses. Currently, aromatic plants are used in pharmaceutical and food industries. One of the most commonly used aromatic plants is thyme. Thyme is a perennial aromatic plant, taxonomically belonging to the genera *Thymus* and *Thymbra*, belonging to the family Lamiaceae. These plants are very abundant in the Mediterranean Region. In this review, we focus on the study of the properties and use of EOs of *Thymbra capitata* (L) Cav. and *Thymus hyemalis* Lange., whose EOs are rich in phenolic monoterpenes. These compounds are responsible for their antioxidant, anti-inflammatory, anticarcinogenic, antibacterial, antifungal, and antiparasitic properties.

Keywords: essential oil, *Thymus hyemalis*, *Thymbra capitata*, aromatic plant, antioxidant, antimicrobial, carvacrol, thymol

1. Introduction

Essential oils (EOs) are volatile odorous compounds, are liquids at room temperature, and are produced by aromatic plants, as a result of their secondary metabolism [1, 2].

In nature, the EOs are stored in the secretory cells, cavities, channels, epidermal cells and trichomes of all the aerial organs of the plants, since they are of vital importance for plant survival, due to their antifungal, antibacterial, and antiviral activities. Also, they provide plants protection against herbivores and allow plants to compete with other plants, acting as allelopathic compounds. In addition, they are involved in pollination, attracting insects which favor the dispersal of seeds and pollen [3].

On the other hand, aromatic plants which produce these EOs have been used since ancient times to treat diseases, due to their healing properties. In fact, there are studies that claim that already in Ancient Egypt (2000 BC), these compounds were used as medicinal remedies, beauty products, and in religious rituals. Likewise, Hippocrates (460–377 BC), the father of medicine, studied and documented the properties of 300 aromatic plants, confirming the use of EOs in Ancient Greece. The Romans also showed great interest in the fragrance and properties of the EOs. Dioscorides, a Greek physician and botanist, described in Ancient Rome more than 500 aromatic plants and their EOs, in his book *De Materia Medica* [4]. In the tenth century, the Arabs also began to extract the EOs and use them in medicine. The use of EOs began to expand due to their pleasant fragrances, and at the end of the twelfth century, they began to be used in Europe. Their popularity was such that when the bubonic plague reached England in the mid-fourteenth century, it was ordered to burn aromatic plants in the streets, to fight the infection. At the beginning of the eighteenth century, EOs were already used to treat many diseases.

In the nineteenth century, EO composition was investigated [5]. It is now known that the major components of EOs are synthesized from three biosynthetic pathways: the mevalonic acid pathway, active in the cytosol, and the methyl erythritol phosphate pathway, active in the chloroplast, both of which lead to the biosynthesis of terpenes. A third route is the shikimic acid pathway, responsible for the biosynthesis of phenylpropanoid compounds [6]. EOs of terpene nature are synthesized from isopentenyl pyrophosphate and its isomer dimethylallyl pyrophosphate, which give rise to geranyl diphosphate, precursor of monoterpenes, and farnesyl diphosphate, precursor of sesquiterpenes, as shown in **Figure 1**. Among the numerous compounds present in the EOs derived from this biosynthetic pathway, thymol and carvacrol (isomers) stand out due to the numerous properties that are granted to them. As seen in **Figure 2**, both are phenolic monoterpenes synthesized from p-cymene, whose precursor is γ-terpinene [7].

Thymol and carvacrol are usually found in thyme EOs. On the other hand, compounds such as alcohols, aldehydes, ketones, esters, and, less frequently, carboxylic acids, as well as aromatic compounds such as phenolic ethers and aromatic esters are also present, although in a significantly lower proportion than the previous ones [6]. The properties of the EOs are mainly attributed to the major compounds, thymol and carvacrol; however it has been observed that these compounds can interact with the minority compounds, causing synergistic or antagonistic effects, thus influencing the properties of the EO [8]. In addition, the chemical composition varies according to environmental and genetic factors, influencing the phenological stage in which the harvest is made on the quality and quantity of the EO [9, 10]. The high variability occurs even within the same species, there being different major compounds among the specimens of the populations, which gives rise to the existence of different chemotypes [11].

Nowadays, many of the active ingredients used in the development of both traditional and modern drugs are extracted from plant species [12]. For the extraction of the EO, the technique most often used is the hydrodistillation, which consists of submerging fragments of the aromatic plant in boiling water, and so, the volatile compounds are dragged with the vapor, arriving at a condenser which separates them, and thus, the EO is obtained. Other conventional techniques such as steam distillation or extraction with volatile solvents as well as hydrodistillation by microwaves or extraction by supercritical fluids can be used [4]. After extracting, EOs can be analyzed by gas chromatography and mass spectrophotometry (GC–MS). GC allows the separation of the components of a complex mixture from the EO, and the MS serves for the identification of the individual components, already separated [13].

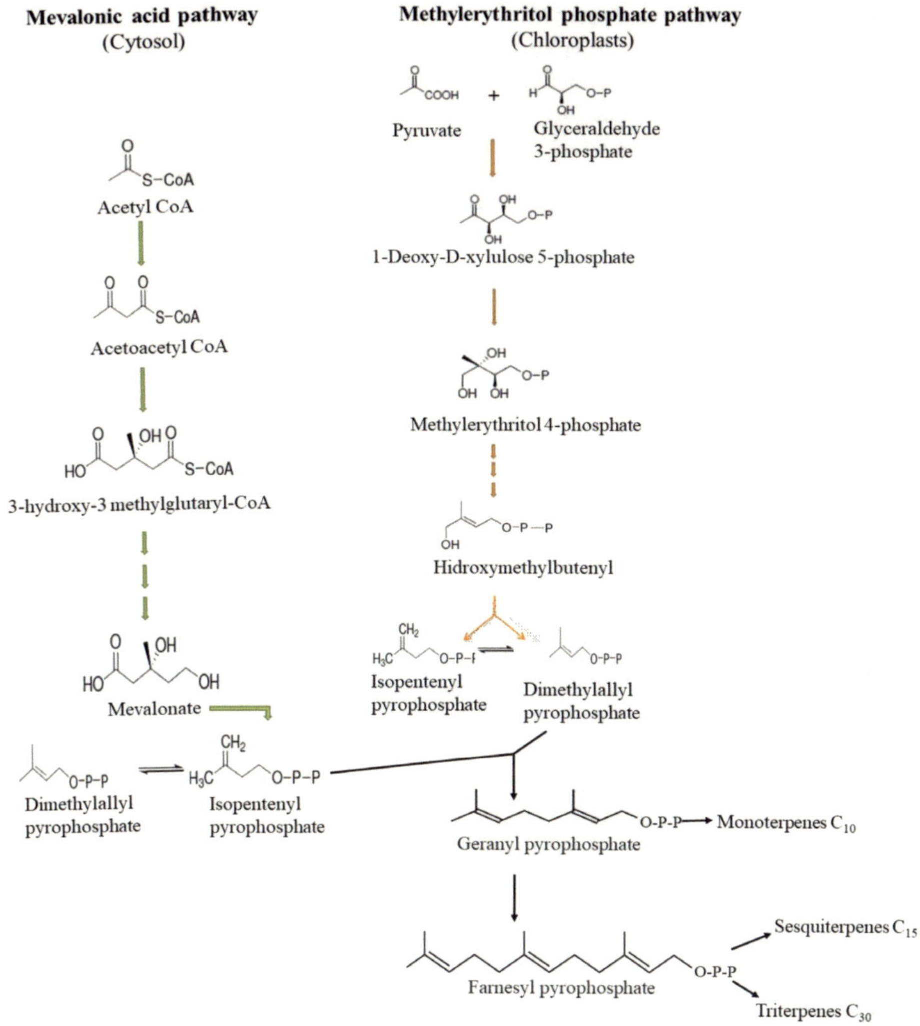

Figure 1.
Biosynthetic pathways responsible for the biosynthesis of the compounds present in the EOs.

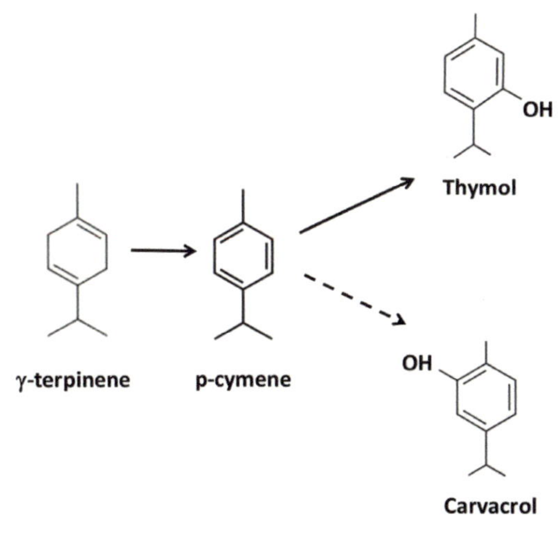

Figure 2.
Thymol and carvacrol chemical structure and their precursors.

Interest in EOs has skyrocketed in recent times. The demand for "natural" products increases year after year, and aromatic plants and EOs are becoming part of daily life. Likewise, more and more people are investigating the use of compounds obtained from plant extracts in medicine, such is the case of the EOs of many aromatic plants such as lavender (*Lavandula angustifolia*), eucalyptus (*Eucalyptus globulus*), or mint (*Mentha piperita*), which are being investigated for their neuroprotective effects [14]. Others such as EOs from oregano (*Origanum spp.*) are studied for their antioxidant and antibacterial activities [15].

It is estimated that more than 250,000 hectares are currently used to produce about 250 different plant extracts and, so on, different EOs, so they have a high socioeconomic importance in the places where they are produced, being generally rural areas in developing countries. These EOs are often used in the food industry as well as in other products of daily use such as bath gels, soaps, detergents, oral care products and body lotions. They are also widely used in aromatherapy (International Trade Center 2014). This justifies that, on a global level, 45,000 tons of EOs are produced annually, which implies an investment of more than 600 million euros, according to a study carried out by the Ministry of Agriculture of France. The main exporters are China, the USA, Brazil, EU countries, India, and Indonesia, and the largest imports are Switzerland, the USA, EU countries, Japan, and Canada [16].

In the industry of the EOs, one of the aromatic plants with greater use is thyme. Thyme is a small shrub and perennial aromatic plant, belonging taxonomically to the genera *Thymus* and *Thymbra*, of the family *Lamiaceae*, which includes 220 genera with plants such as mint, peppermint, basil, oregano, or pennyroyal, known throughout the world [17]. Thyme is very abundant in the Mediterranean Region. In the Iberian Peninsula, there is a high number of endemism, and it is common to find them in groups of thickets commonly known as "tomillares" [18]. Spain is one of the main suppliers of thyme worldwide [19], being the provinces with higher production Almeria, Murcia, and Granada, although it is also important in other areas of Andalusia, Castilla-La Mancha, and other provinces of interior, as Teruel [20].

Within the Region of Murcia, we found several species of thyme, two of them being of special relevance, both for their properties and for their environmental situation [18]: (1) *Thymbra capitata* (L.) Cav., commonly known as the Andalusian thyme, has a compact and stiff, fairly branched shrubby appearance, with pink flowers arranged in pineapple-shaped heads and leaves that are linear, glandular, and fleshy-looking, with a flat margin (**Figure 3**) [21]. (2) *Thymus hyemalis* Lange, commonly known as purple thyme or winter thyme, since the flowering stage

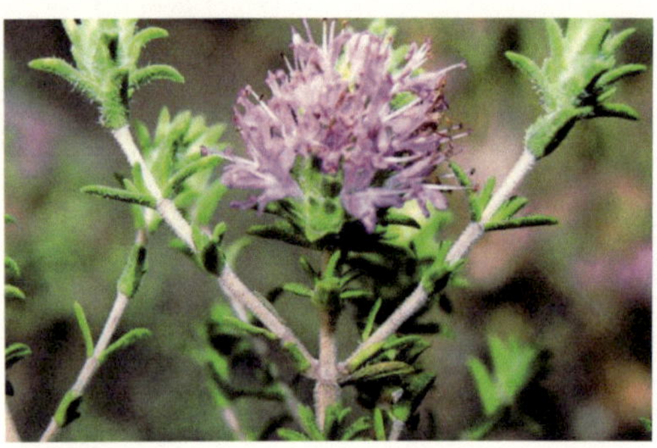

Figure 3.
T. capitata *inflorescence, characteristical disposal, and leaf morphology.*

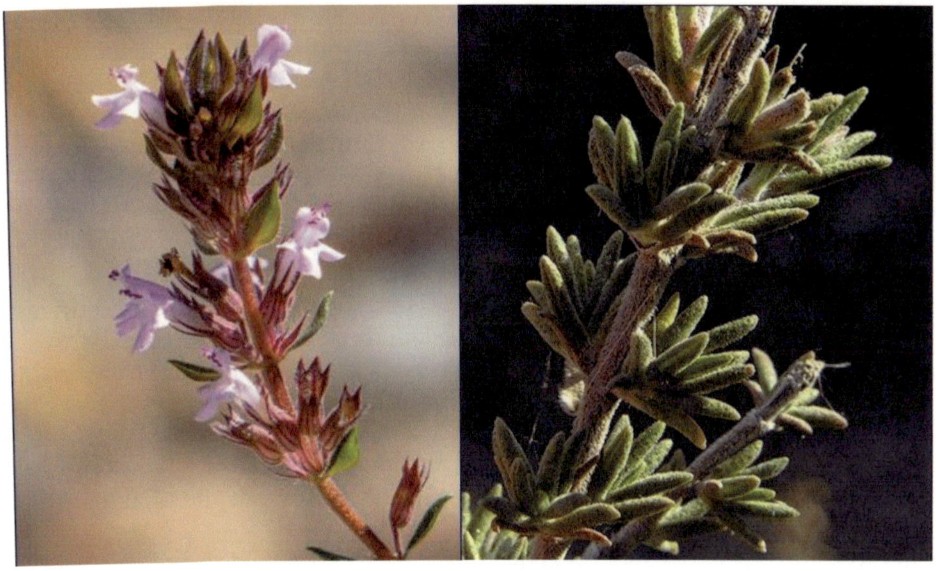

Figure 4.
T. hyemalis *inflorescence (left), characteristical disposal, and leaf morphology (right).*

occurs in this season of the year, is a much branched woody shrub whose flowers have a pink corolla and a calyx with ciliated teeth, with leaves that are of small size, linear, and with revolute margin [22] (**Figure 4**).

This work focuses on these two species, due to the fact that *T. capitata*, a species of Mediterranean distribution, is found in the Region of Murcia in a retrograde situation and *T. hyemalis* is an endemic species from southeastern Spain, being mainly found in Murcia and Almería [18]. In addition, the properties and the possible uses of their EOs are the aims of this review.

2. Bioactive compounds of *T. capitata* EO

According to several studies, the EO of *T. capitata* is characterized by its high chemical homogeneity. Russo et al. [23], in an experiment carried out with wild populations of *T. capitata* in Calabria (Italy), observed that all the collected specimens, despite having grown under different environmental conditions, had a very similar chemical composition and all the specimens were of chemotype carvacrol (81.5–78.4%). A relatively high percentage of *p*-cymene, γ-terpinene, and β-caryophyllene were also found in these specimens. In addition, it has been observed that the percentages of *p*-cymene and γ-terpinene decreased when the percentage of carvacrol increased, which indicated that both compounds were its precursors [24]. Saija et al. [25], studying the chemical composition of this EO found that, all the wild specimens of *T. capitata* analyzed were of chemotype carvacrol. These results agree with studies conducted by Miguel et al. [9, 26, 27], where the major component was carvacrol, regardless of both the part of the plant used and the state of development. Likewise, Tuttolomondo et al. [28], in Sicily (Italy), found 38 compounds, being the most representative α-pinene, myrcene, α-terpinene, *p*-cymene, γ-terpinene, borneol, β-caryophyllene and carvacrol (67.4–79.5%), being the 13 biotypes studied of carvacrol chemotype. These results suggest that there is no polymorphism in the EO of *T. capitata*. However, other studies are contradictory to the results mentioned above, showing the existence of three different chemotypes for *T. capitata*. In this sense, Miceli et al. [29] found 75 components and the majority being carvacrol and thymol, which, in all cases, constituted more than 50% of the composition of EO, followed by γ-terpinene, borneol, and *p*-cymene, when the chemical composition of the EO of *T. capitata* specimens were analyzed in flowering stage. The analysis of the compounds found in this EO revealed that there was a direct correlation between myrcene, α-terpinene, and γ-terpinene, whose concentrations decreased as the thymol concentration increased. An inverse relationship between linalool and myrcene was also observed. Thus, the analysis of the compounds presents in the EO of the specimens studied revealed that there were three distinct chemotypes: thymol, carvacrol, and thymol/carvacrol, the most common being those of chemotype thymol. For the first two chemotypes, a negative correlation was observed between thymol and carvacrol, so when one of the components was majority, the other was at low concentration. The thymol /carvacrol chemotype resulted from the crossing between the specimens with the two previous chemotypes. In short, independently of the chemotype, it was observed that the content of monoterpenes reached 78% of the total of compounds present in the EO of *T. capitata* [29].

In this sense, the experiments carried out by [10] confirmed the existence of these three chemotypes, which supports the hypothesis that *T. capitata* has a high polymorphism in the EO composition. To carry out these experiments, specimens grown in areas at different temperatures and degrees of humidity were used. As a result of this experiment, it was observed that those of carvacrol chemotype only appeared under conditions of high temperatures and low humidity. On the other hand, an experiment was carried out in which nine specimens were used, collected from three different areas, to later be cultivated under the same controlled climatic conditions. The results showed that the specimens maintained the chemotype that they originally presented, which is determined genetically, and did not change in the absence of climatic variations. These data suggest that the chemical composition of the EO is determined by the genetic endowment of the specimen and the different chemotypes are distributed according to the environmental conditions of the area in which they are cultivated [30].

Finally, in relation to other components found in smaller proportion (such as geraniol, camphor, or β-caryophyllene, among others), there is a high variability between populations and even within the same population [24, 31]. This variability can influence the bioactivity of *T. capitata* EO, which does not only depend on the majority component but also depends on the synergistic and antagonistic interactions that occur among all the phenolic and non-phenolic components [9, 25–27].

3. Bioactive compounds of *T. hyemalis* EO

In a study conducted by [32], it was observed that *T. hyemalis* EO had a high heterogeneity, there being three different chemotypes: thymol, thymol/linalool, and carvacrol. The main components for the thymol chemotype were thymol (43%) followed by p-cymene (16%) and γ-terpinene (8.4%). For the thymol/linalool chemotype, the major compounds were linalool (16.6%), thymol (16%), γ-terpinene (9.8%), 1–8-cineol (5.4%), borneol (4.7%), and verbenone (4.8%). Finally, the carvacrol chemotype was characterized by a majority composition of carvacrol (40.1%), *p*-cymene (19.8%), borneol (5.0%), and thymol (2.9%).

The variability in the chemical composition of *T. hyemalis* EO may be related to seasonal variations [33, 34] as well as to the edapho-climatic factors [35].

One of the studies that supports the previous statement were carried out by Jordán et al. [36], where it was observed that, in the case of thymol chemotype, the synthesis of this major compound occurred during the flowering/fruit ripening stage. The precursors of thymol, γ-terpinene, and *p*-cymene (**Figure 1**) were at their maximum concentration during the flowering stage. Therefore, between the stage of flowering and that of the beginning of fruit maturation, the composition of the EO of *T. hyemalis* reached its highest quality. This phenological stage coincides with winter, being recommendable to harvest the specimens in this season of the year. However, according to this study, it is also possible to obtain a high thymol content in the *T. hyemalis* EO during the spring season, but to achieve this, it is necessary to increase the irrigation, a condition that is not always achieved in arid and semiarid regions. In contrast to these results, Cabo et al. [33] proposed that August was the best time to harvest because the *T. hyemalis* EO contained a high concentration of 1,8-cineol in specimens collected during different phases of the vegetative cycle of *T. hyemalis*. These results seem to indicate the existence of a 1,8-cineol chemotype, with a very low concentration of thymol and carvacrol.

Finally, similar to the results of *T. capitata,* it should be noted that although the phenolic compounds, thymol and carvacrol, are mainly responsible for the bioactivity of the EO, the existence of synergistic or antagonistic effects between these phenolic components and other minor compounds (alcohols, other terpenoids, ketones, etc.) of *T. hyemalis* EO has been observed, which are essential for the quality of this EO [32].

4. Bioactivity of *T. capitata* EO

4.1 Antioxidant activity

It has been observed that the EO of *T. capitata* shows a potent antioxidant activity due to its high content of phenols (thymol or carvacrol) [37]. This statement is supported by Aazza et al. [38], when compared with the antioxidant activity of several thyme species. The results showed a higher antioxidant activity in EO rich in phenolic monoterpenes, like those of *Thymus caespititius* Brot. and *T. capitata*.

This antioxidant capacity has been widely researched in order to prevent lipid oxidation during the storage of vegetable oils for culinary use, such as olive or sunflower. Likewise, Miguel et al. [26] showed that *T. capitata* EO, rich in carvacrol, avoided the lipid oxidation of sunflower oil and even turned out to be a more potent antioxidant than butylated hydroxytoluene (BHT), a synthetic antioxidant commonly used in the food industry. In addition, it has been seen that by isolating the carvacrol from the EO, this one by itself showed an antioxidant activity like EO, indicating an absence of synergistic or antagonistic effects due to the interaction between the different components of the EO. However, when the antioxidant activity of the EO of *T. capitata* was tested on the lipid oxidation of olive oil, it was observed that the EO was less potent than BHT [27, 39]. This low antioxidant capacity is also evident in the studies conducted by Saavedra et al. [40], in which it was observed that *T. capitata* EO did not help to avoid the oxidation of olive oil during storage and even increased the peroxidation levels, which indicated a greater number of oxidation products.

Another study conducted by Miguel et al. [9] on the lipid oxidation of peanut and sunflower oils showed a low antioxidant activity of *T. capitata* EO compared to two synthetic antioxidants, hydroxybutylanisole (BHA) and BHT, as well as a low effectiveness in elimination of free radicals compared to BHT, which contradicts the previous results found in sunflower oil. In addition, when comparing the EO of *T. capitata* with those of other species of the family Lamiaceae (*T. mastichina* and *T. camphoratus*), rich in *p*-cymene-2,3-diol, it was observed that the EO of *T. capitata*, rich in carvacrol, had a lower antioxidant activity than those of these two species. These results could be due to the differences found at the time of harvest, since, in this study, the *T. capitata* specimens were collected in the vegetative phase, while in the studies that demonstrated an important antioxidant activity for the EO of *T. capitata*, the specimens were collected during the flowering phase.

On the other hand, Galego et al. [41] carried out a study on the antioxidant capacity of EOs extracted from *T. capitata*, *Origanum vulgare* L., *T. mastichina*, and *Calamintha baetica* Boiss & Reut. For this, the antioxidant activity was determined using modified thiobarbituric acid (TBARS), which consists of the formation of a pink pigment produced by the reaction of thiobarbituric acid with malondialdehyde, a product of lipid peroxidation. Their results indicated that *T. capitata* and *O. vulgare* had the highest antioxidant activity, like BHT and BHA, but although they were effective in eliminating free radicals, at low concentrations, they did not become as effective as BHT and BHA.

In addition, it was observed that the antioxidant capacity of the EO of *T. capitata* was higher than that of the EO of *T. mastichina* and *C. baetica*, since the composition of the EO of these species was lower in phenolic compounds than the EO of *T. capitata*.

Faleiro et al. [15] also used the TBARS method to observe the effectiveness of the EO of *T. capitata* against the lipid oxidation of the egg yolk. Their results showed that, at high concentrations, EO could be as effective as synthetic antioxidants, BHA and BHT.

It should be noted that the antioxidant activity of *T. capitata* EO has not only been investigated in the food industry. In this sense, Hortigón-Vinagre et al. [42] studied the ability of this EO to prevent the cell death of cardiomyocytes in neonatal rats treated with 4-hydroxy-2-nonenal, a compound that induces lipid peroxidation in these cells. The results showed that at low concentrations (less than 40 ppm), the EO of *T. capitata* prevented the loss of membrane potential of the mitochondria and decreased the levels of reactive oxygen species (ROS), preventing the death of cardiomyocytes. However, concentrations higher than the mentioned one caused cell death, since they were toxic for the cells. In addition, this toxicity can be used as antiproliferative activity in in vitro experiments, since the EO extracted from fruits of *T. capitata* inhibited the growth of cells isolated from cervical cancer (HeLa). Likewise, the EO extracted from flowers and fruits of this species inhibited the growth of histiocytosis cells (U937) [30] and tumor cells responsible for acute monocytic leukemia (THP-1) [37].

4.2 Antibacterial activity

The antibacterial activity of the EO of *T. capitata* as well as its main component, carvacrol, was demonstrated against *Gardnerella vaginalis* by Machado et al. [43, 44]. The EO of *T. capitata* showed a potent activity against *G. vaginalis*, which was evidenced by the low minimum inhibitory concentration (MIC) (0.16 μL/mL) and the minimum lethal concentration (MLC) (0.16–0.31 μL/mL).

This antibacterial activity of *T. capitata* EO has also been observed against *Listeria monocytogenes*, the bacteria responsible for listeriosis, in a study conducted by Faleiro et al. [15].

In addition, Delgado-Adámez et al. [30] showed that the EO extracted from both flowers and fruits of *T. capitata* had a high efficacy against *Listeria innocua* (Gram+), at concentrations higher than 0.01% (v/v), and *Escherichia coli* (Gram−), at concentrations above 0.1% (v/v). Also, Karampoula et al. [45] showed the antibacterial effectiveness of the EO of *T. capitata* in hydrosol (a complex mixture of 24 components, which came from hydrodistillation of the plant, where the major compound was carvacrol). This antibacterial activity was studied against planktonic cells and biofilms of *Salmonella typhimurium*. The biofilms formed by the bacteria showed a slightly higher resistance to the planktonic cells, but in general, hydrosol was effective as antibacterial agent. In fact, when comparing this hydrosol with benzalkonium chloride, a commonly used synthetic antibacterial, it was observed that the hydrosol from *T. capitata* EO was much more effective as bactericide, since in order for benzalkonium chloride to show the same results as the hydrosol on planktonic cells and biofilms of *S. typhimurium*, a 200 times higher concentration was needed.

4.3 Antifungal activity

According to Salgueiro et al. [46], the EO of 22 specimens of *T. capitata* carvacrol chemotype (60–66%), with high percentages of p-cymene (6–7.5%) and γ-terpinene (8.2–9.5%), was effective as a natural antifungal agent against *Candida* spp., *Aspergillus* spp., and some species of dermatophytes (*Trichophyton rubrum*, *T. mentagrophytes*, *Microsporum canis*, and *M. gypseum*), and its effect was mainly due to the generation of lesions on the membrane surface of the microorganism.

These results agree with Palmeira-de-Oliveira et al. [47, 48], whose studies demonstrated that the EO of *T. capitata*, rich in carvacrol (75%), showed a great antifungal potential on biomass of *Candida* spp. and on preformed biofilms, since, at concentrations close to MIC (0.32 μL/mL), it caused the inhibition of its metabolism by up to 50%.

In the case of biofilms, when the concentration of the EO doubled the MIC, a decrease of 80% of its metabolism was observed. Antifungal activity of the EO of *T. capitata* was also compared with the classic antifungal agents amphotericin B and fluconazole, proving to be even more effective in some of the fungi studied.

Likewise, it has been observed that carvacrol or *p*-cymene isolated from the EO of *T. capitata* by themselves showed antifungal capacity. Therefore, this EO, or its isolated components, could be used for the treatment of mucocutaneous candidiasis and dermatophytosis. In this sense, the EO of *T. capitata* could be used alone or together with other antifungal components used so far [46, 47], as in the case of the association of the EO of *T capitata* with chitosan or chitosan in hydrogel, whose antifungal activity has been demonstrated in in vitro studies. The mechanism of action of this hydrogel has been studied by confocal microscopy, observing the interaction of this formula with the cell wall of *Candida* spp. [46].

On the other hand, Russo et al. [23] observed that the EO of *T. capitata* carvacrol chemotype had an antifungal effect at a concentration of 250 ppm against *Sclerotium cepivorum*, a fungus responsible for white rot in garlic, onion, and leek crops. These authors suggested that the EO of *T. capitata* could be used as a natural antifungal, for its plant origin, not being harmful to the environment. In addition, it would be difficult to develop resistance in the fungus, due to the high chemical complexity of this oil.

4.4 Antiparasitic activity

Machado et al. [22] analyzed the antiparasitic activity of EOs rich in phenolic compounds of the species *T. capitata*, *O. virens* (Hoffmanns & Link), *T. zygis* subsp. *Sylvestris* (Hoffmanns & Link) Cout., and *Lippia graveolens* Kunth against *Giardia* spp. All EOs, including that of *T. capitata*, decreasing the viability of the parasite; altering its morphology, membrane permeability, and internal organization; and inhibiting its growth, as well as its adhesion capacity, which is essential for the parasite, to be able to bind to the intestine and not be eliminated by peristalsis. EOs blocked this adhesion from the first hours of exposure, not being more than 10% of cells able to adhere after 7 hours of treatment. In addition, by affecting membrane permeability, they caused swelling in the cells and alterations in the cytoplasm, which ultimately leads to cell death. Therefore, these EOs could be used as an alternative treatment for giardiasis, since they are not toxic to mammalian cells.

5. Bioactivity of *T. hyemalis* EO

5.1 Antioxidant activity

Several studies have shown the antioxidant activity of *T. hyemalis* EO. In this sense, Ocaña and Reglero [49] analyzed the antioxidant properties of the EO of *T. hyemalis*, *T. zygis*, and *Thymus vulgaris* L. on a cellular model of inflammation/atherogenesis, in which human macrophages, derived from THP-1 cells, were used. These cells were incubated with EOs of the different Thymus species. The expression of inflammatory (TNF-α, IL-1B and IL-6) and anti-inflammatory (IL-10) mediators was determined. The results showed that the production of inflammatory mediators took place and the production of the anti-inflammatory mediator IL-10 increased in the presence of EOs of any of the three species of Thymus (being *T. hyemalis* the one that had less activity). This effect is due to the antioxidant capacity of these EOs, which in turn is responsible for the anti-inflammatory activity observed in this test.

On the other hand, Jennan et al. [50] compared the activity of the EO of *T. hyemalis* with that of the EO of *Thymus bleicherianus* Pomel, measuring its capacity to eliminate the free radical 1,1-diphenyl-2-picrilhydracil, observing a greater antioxidant activity in the EO of *T. bleicherianus*. The activity of EO of *T. hyemalis* was also compared with that of BHT, the synthetic compound being a more potent antioxidant. These results suggested that, although the *T. hyemalis* EO is a good antioxidant, it is not as good as the EO of other *Thymus* species.

5.2 Antibacterial activity

Rota et al. [32] conducted a study on the antimicrobial activity of EOs from several thyme species, specifically, *T. hyemalis*, *T. zygis*, and *T. vulgaris*. The EO activity was tested against the pathogenic microorganisms *E. coli*, *L. monocytogenes*, *S. typhimurium*, *Shigella flexneri*, *Shigella sonnei*, *Staphylococcus aureus*, *and Yersinia enterocolitica*. The results showed that the antimicrobial activity seemed to be related to the content of phenolic compounds, specifically thymol and carvacrol. EOs that showed the greatest antimicrobial effectiveness were *T. hyemalis* (thymol and carvacrol chemotypes, in this order), *T. zygis* (thymol), and *T. vulgaris* (thymol). These results coincided with those found by Jennan et al. [50] which suggested that *T. hyemalis* EO affected survival and inhibited the growth of bacteria Gram+ and Gram−.

Some microorganisms, such as *S. typhimurium*, *Y. enterocolitica*, *S. flexneri*, *L. monocytogenes*, and *S. aureus*, showed a high sensitivity to EOs from *T. hyemalis* (thymol and thymol/linalool chemotypes), so a high concentration of them to be effective was not necessary. In other cases, such as *E. coli*, the presence of a high concentration of carvacrol or thymol was essential to observe a potent antibacterial activity. In addition, it has been observed that the greater the richness and variety of minority components, the greater the effectiveness of EO against microorganisms [32].

Tepe et al. [51] also investigated the in vitro antimicrobial activity of *T. hyemalis* EO (carvacrol chemotype), which turned out to be a potent bactericide at low

Microorganisms	MIC Commercially available essential oil component		
	Thymol	Carvacrol	p-cymene
Staphylococcus aureus	1.95	0.48	250.00
Bacillus cereus	0.97	0.24	250.00
Enterobacter aerogenes	0.97	1.95	250.00
Escherichia coli	1.95	0.48	250.00
Klebsiella pneumoniae	1.95	3.90	250.00
Proteus mirabilis	1.95	1.95	250.00
Pseudomonas aeruginosa	15.62	7.81	250.00
Candida albicans	0.97	0.24	15.62

Table 1.
Antibacterial and antifungal activity of the three major components found in T. hyemalis *EO [51].*

concentrations (31.2 mg/mL) against *Bacillus cereus* and *Bacillus subtilis*. In addition, it also inhibited the growth of *Enterococcus faecalis* and *S. aureus*, although at higher concentrations (62.5 mg/mL). They also studied the antimicrobial activity of isolated carvacrol, which showed a potent activity against *B. cereus*, showing inhibition of bacterial growth with a MIC of 0.24 mg/mL. It also showed activity against *E. coli*, although at higher concentrations (**Table 1**).

This activity of carvacrol was compared with the antibacterial activity of thymol, the second most important component of *T. hyemalis* EO (carvacrol chemotype). The results obtained suggested that thymol was a good bactericide, but not as much as carvacrol. However, when the isolated precursor of carvacrol (p-cymene) was used, no antimicrobial activity was observed. Also, neither the *T. hyemalis* EO nor the isolated carvacrol was effective against *Klebsiella pneumoniae*, *Pseudomonas aeruginosa*, *Pseudomonas fluorescens*, *and L. monocytogenes*.

5.3 Antifungal activity

Tepe et al. [51] demonstrated the antifungal activity of *T. hyemalis* EO against *C. albicans*, which inhibited its growth at a MIC of 62.50 mg/mL. This activity was also measured using carvacrol, thymol, and p-cymene, major components of *T. hyemalis* EO. Carvacrol inhibited the growth of the fungus at a MIC of 0.24 mg/mL, while p-cymene needed high concentrations to begin to inhibit fungal growth. Thymol was also a good antifungal against *C. albicans*, although not as good as carvacrol, since the MIC turned out to be 0.97 mg/mL.

6. Discussion

In general, all the data together show that *T. capitata* and *T. hyemalis* are two important sources of EOs, which have different types of bioactivity, being of great interest for human health as well as for food and cosmetics, due to their antifungal, antibacterial, and antioxidant properties.

According to the literature reviewed, the biological activity found in the EOs is clearly related to the chemical composition of them. As regards the *T. capitata* EO, there are some controversies about its homogeneity. Several studies confirm the existence of a single chemotype in this species, determined by its major component, carvacrol [9, 23–28]. However, other studies support the existence of three chemotypes: thymol, carvacrol, and thymol/carvacrol, resulting in a crossover from the previous two [10, 29]. Regarding *T. hyemalis*, there is no doubt about the heterogeneity of its EO, being the chemotypes: thymol, thymol/linalool, and carvacrol [32].

For both species (*T. capitata* and *T. hyemalis*), the reason for these differences in the chemical composition of their EOs extracted from different specimens could be due both to the genetic endowment of the plants and to the influence of climatic and edaphic conditions of their habitat. In fact, the influence of climate on the composition of EOs has also been described for other species within the genus Thymus, such as *T. zygis* and *T. piperella*. In general, carvacrol-rich chemotypes have been associated with arid climates and high areas. However, thymol-rich chemotypes have higher water requirements than the carvacrol chemotypes [11, 52].

Likewise, the moment in which the specimens are harvested influences the composition of EOs, since it varies throughout the life cycle of these plants, affecting their bioactivities. In fact, in *T. capitata*, the highest content of phenolic monoterpenes occurs during the flowering stage, exhibiting greater antioxidant activity at this time. This coincides with what has been demonstrated for other thyme species, such as *T. vulgaris* [53]. For this reason, it is recommended to collect them during this stage, achieving the highest qualities of this EO. Regarding *T. hyemalis*, there is controversy about the best time to harvest. Extensively works support that it is better to collect the specimens in winter, between the flowering stage and the beginning stage of fruit ripening. However, other authors propose that the best month to harvest is August, since, during this month, there is a high content of 1,8-cineol in the EO. These results point to the possible existence of a 1,8-cineol chemotype, but further studies would be necessary to confirm this hypothesis. If this compound is a major component in *T. hyemalis*, the exploitation of this chemotype at an industrial level could be interesting, since it has been shown that 1,8-cineol has anti-inflammatory and analgesic properties [54]. It has also been observed that it can act as a natural insecticide in certain plant species of the *Myrtaceae* family [55].

On the other hand, the results show that in the absence of environmental variations, the different chemotypes are genetically determined. This has been observed for the EO of other medicinal plants, such as *Lupinus argenteus* Pursh and *Piper methysticum* G. Forst, whose mutations in a few genes influence the biosynthetic pathways which promote the greater or lesser accumulation of one or another compound, giving rise to different chemotypes [56, 57].

Regarding the antioxidant activity, the results indicate that it depends on the concentration. The EO of *T. capitata* (carvacrol chemotype) is effective at high concentration to avoid lipid oxidation of egg yolk and sunflower oil and may be even more effective than BHA and BHT. However, this is only possible if *T. capitata* specimens have been harvested during the flowering stage [7, 9].

This is due, in large part, to the fact that the antioxidant activity of EO (as well as the rest of activities) does not depend only on the majority component but also depends on the synergistic or antagonistic interactions of the majority component with other minority components, which according to the phenological stage will be different [58]. However, in the literature reviewed, some authors indicate the absence of these interactions because isolated carvacrol has been shown to have activity on its own [27, 39]. However, the EO of *T. capitata* did not prove to be a good antioxidant for olive oil. This is the difference between sunflower oil and olive oil. This difference can be due to the different compositions of fatty acids in both oils, being the most effective in sunflower oil (rich in linoleic) than in olive (rich in oleic) [39].

On the other hand, both EOs extracted from *T. capitata* specimens and *T. hyemalis*, at low concentrations, have antioxidant activity, which gives them anti-inflammatory properties, which could be used for the treatment of chronic inflammatory diseases. However, at high concentrations, EOs of these species show oxidant activity, which could be toxic to the cells and so inhibit their proliferation. This effect of EOs on cell proliferation is of great interest since they could be used as potent anticancer agents [49].

Regarding their antibacterial activity, EOs have shown a potent bactericidal effect against a large number of Gram+ and Gram- species. In this sense, EO of *T. capitata* could be used for the treatment of bacterial vaginosis together with chitosan in hydrogel; this could be a good alternative to treatment with antibiotics, which usually provoke resistance. In addition, it has been observed that EOs are well tolerated by the beneficial flora, since it is not damaged [43, 44].

Likewise, both EOs from *T. capitata* and *T. hyemalis* (all the chemotypes, although the most effective is the thymol chemotype) are useful against *L. monocytogenes*, so they could be used in the food industry to avoid contamination due to this bacterium [15].

In relation to the antifungal activity, it has been demonstrated for the EO of *T. capitata* (carvacrol chemotype) against *Candida* spp., *Aspergillus* spp., and some species of dermatophytes (*Trichophyton rubrum*, *T. mentagrophytes*, *Microsporum canis*, and *M. gypseum*). This EO has also shown activity against the intestinal parasite *Giardia* spp. This fact suggests that it could be used for the treatment of giardiasis together with other compounds such as chitosan.

In addition, the *T. hyemalis* EO (carvacrol chemotype) and carvacrol by itself also showed effectiveness against *C. albicans*. However, it has not been demonstrated for its precursor, p-cymene. Although the antimicrobial activity depends on the presence of carvacrol, it is believed that p-cymene acts synergistically with carvacrol, helping to destabilize the membrane of these microorganisms.

Currently, the trade and use of thyme EOs is more focused on species such as *T. vulgaris*. This species has been widely used in aromatherapy and natural medicine for some years, as a hot poultice that relieves the pain of cystitis and renal colic, due to its analgesic properties, and in the form of vapors and inhalations for asthma and colds, among other conditions of the respiratory system. It is also used as a natural disinfectant, due to its antiseptic power. Its antimicrobial, antioxidant, and anticancer properties have been widely studied. However, the information reviewed here indicates that these two species, *T. capitata* and *T. hyemalis*, could be a very important source of economic resources, due to their properties, since they can be exploited by the pharmaceutical, food, livestock, and agricultural industries, its conservation being fundamental in the ecosystems where they are found.

Finally, in relation to the mechanism of action by which EOs have their different effects, it is not clear. It is known that all the activities mentioned are dependent on the concentration at which they are used. As we have seen throughout this work, the results vary depending on the dose of EO used. With regard to the antifungal and antibacterial activity, the EO acts by affecting the membrane permeability of the pathogen. At high concentrations, the EO denatures the proteins, whereas if the concentration is low, the enzymatic activity related to the production of energy is affected.

It has also been observed that, in the case of *Sclerotium cepivorum* Berk, in the presence of monoterpenes, its lipid composition is modified, the cell membrane is altered, and lipid peroxidation is increased, so that these compounds are toxic for the cells. Therefore, these EOs, rich in monoterpenes, could be used to treat crops affected by diseases caused by fungi, such as white rot, which would be a great economic benefit, since it would avoid large agricultural losses. However, it would be necessary to carry out further studies on the mechanism of action of the compounds present in the EOs, specifically the content of monoterpenes in both

T. capitata and *T. hyemalis*. In addition, most of the studies reviewed were carried out in in vitro experiments, so to ensure the potential of these EOs, it would be necessary to study their properties in vivo.

7. Conclusion

T. capitata and *T. hyemalis* EOs are rich in phenolic monoterpenes (carvacrol and thymol), which are associated with antioxidant, antifungal, antibacterial, or antiparasitic properties. These EOs, due to their properties, can be used in pharmaceutical, food, livestock, agricultural, and pharmaceutical industries, being a potential source of economic resources. However, climate, edaphic factors, and genetics influence the chemical composition of these EOs. The high homogeneity of *T. capitata* EOs in climates with high temperatures and low humidity (carvacrol chemotype) can be an important economic resource of easy exploitation in arid and semiarid regions.

Acknowledgements

This work was supported by the CDTI (No. IDI-20150891).

Conflict of interest

The authors declare that there are no conflicts of interest.

Author details

Ana Belén Sabater-Jara, María Pina Funes, María Angeles Pedreño and Sarai Belchí-Navarro*
University of Murcia, Murcia, Spain

*Address all correspondence to: saraibn@um.es

References

[1] Lawerence BM, Reynolds RJ. Progress in essential oils. Perfumer and Flavorist. 2001;**26**:44-52

[2] Opender K, Suresh W, Dhaliwal GS. Essential oils as green pesticides potential and constraints. Biopesticides International. 2008;**4**(1):63-84

[3] Croteau R, Kutchan TM, Lewis NG. Natural products (secondary metabolites). In: Buchanan B, Gruissem W, Jones R, editors. Biochemistry and Molecular Biology of Plants. American Society of Plant Physiologists; 2000. pp. 1250-1318

[4] Kubeczka KH. History and sources of essential oils research. In: Can Baser KH, Buchbauer G, editors. Handbook of Essential Oils: Science, Technology, and Applications. 2nd ed. Boca Raton: CRC Press; 2015. pp. 5-43

[5] Fletcher JC, Riley MJH. U.S. Patent No. 6,280,751. Washington, DC: U.S. Patent and Trademark Office; 2001

[6] Sell C. Chemistry of essential oils. In: Can Baser KH, Buchbauer G, editors. Handbook of Essential Oils: Science, Technology, and Applications. 2nd ed. Boca Raton: CRC Press; 2010. pp. 121-150

[7] Salas JB, Téllez TR, Alonso MJ, Pardo FM, de los Ángeles Cases Capdevila M, Rodríguez CG. Chemical composition and antioxidant activity of the essential oil of *Thymbra capitata* (L.) Cav. in Spain. Acta Botanica Gallica. 2010;**157**(1):55-63. DOI: 10.1080/12538078.2010.10516189

[8] Savelev S, Okello E, Perry NSL, Wilkins RM, Perry EK. Synergistic and antagonistic interactions of anticholinesterase terpenoids in *Salvia lavandulaefolia* essential oil. Pharmacology Biochemistry and Behavior, Plants and the Central Nervous System. 2003;**75**:661-668. DOI: 10.1016/S0091-3057(03)00125-4

[9] Miguel MG, Falcato-Simões M, Figueiredo AC, Barroso JMG, Pedro LG, Carvalho LM. Evaluation of the antioxidant activity of *Thymbra capitata*, *Thymus mastichina* and *Thymus camphoratus* essential oils. Journal of Food Lipids. 2005;**12**(3):181-197. DOI: 10.1111/j.1745-4522.2005.00015x

[10] Tommasi L, Negro C, Cerfeda A, Nutricati E, Zuccarello V, Bellis LD, et al. Influence of environmental factors on essential oil variability in *Thymbra capitata* (L.) Cav. Growing wild in southern Puglia (Italy). Journal of Essential Oil Research. 2007;**19**(6):572-580. DOI: 10.1080/10412905.2007.9699335

[11] Sáez F. Essential oil variability of *Thymus zygis* growing wild in southeastern Spain. Phytochemistry. 1995;**40**(3):819-825. DOI: 10.1016/0031-9422(95)00347-A

[12] Bawa S, Kumar S, Drabu S, Kumar R. Structural modifications of quinoline-based antimalarial agents: Recent developments. Journal of Pharmacy and Bioallied Sciences. 2010;**2**(2):64-71. DOI: 10.4103/0975-7406.67002

[13] Guzmán ML. Técnicas Espectrometría de masas. Unidad de Espectrometría de Masas. Servicios Centrales de Apoyo a la Investigación. Universidad de Málaga; 2011

[14] Ayaz M, Sadiq A, Junaid M, Ullah F, Subhan F, Ahmed J. Neuroprotective and anti-aging potentials of essential oils from aromatic and medicinal plants. Frontiers in Aging Neuroscience. 2017;**9**:168

[15] Faleiro L, Miguel G, Gomes S, Costa L, Venâncio F, Teixeira A, et al.

Antibacterial and antioxidant activities of essential oils isolated from *Thymbra capitata* L. (Cav.) and *Origanum vulgare* L. Journal of Agricultural and Food Chemistry. 2005;**53**(21):8162-8168. DOI: 10.1021/jf0510079

[16] Verlet N. Overview of the essential oils economy. Acta Horticulturae. 1993;**333**:65-72. DOI: 10.17660/actahortic.1993.333.4

[17] Morales R. Taxonomía de los géneros Thymus (excluida la sección Serpyllum) y Thymbra en la Peninsula Ibérica. Ruizia. 1986;**3**:1-324

[18] Sánchez P, Guerra J, Jiménez J, Cánovas JL, Torrente P. Guía de las plantas aromático-medicinales y otras especies de interés económico del Noreste de la Región de Murcia. Murcia: Integral. Sociedad para el desarrollo rural; 2015

[19] Lawrence B.M & Tucker A.O. 2003. The genus thymus as a source of commercial products. In: Stahl-Biskup E., Sáez F. (eds) Thyme: The Genus Thymus. Taylor & Francis. London: CRC Press; 252-263

[20] Torrente F. El tomillo: Aprovechamiento y cultivo. Hojas divulgadoras. Ministerio de Agricultura y Pesca. Alimentación y Medio Ambiente. Gobierno de España; 1985

[21] Polunin O, Smythies BE. Guía de campo de las flores de España, Portugal y Sudoeste de Francia. Barcelona: Ediciones Omega, S.A.; 2004

[22] Machado M, Dinis AM, Salgueiro L, Cavaleiro C, Custódio JBA, do Céu Sousa M. Anti-giardia activity of phenolic-rich essential oils: effects of *Thymbra capitata*, *Origanum virens*, *Thymus zygis* subsp. sylvestris, and *Lippia graveolens* on trophozoites growth, viability, adherence, and ultrastructure. Parasitology Research. 2010;**106**(5):1205-1215. DOI: 10.1007/s00436-010-1800-7

[23] Russo M, Suraci F, Postorino S, Serra D, Roccotelli A, Agosteo GE. Essential oil chemical composition and antifungal effects on *Sclerotium cepivorum* of *Thymus capitatus* wild populations from Calabria, southern Italy. Revista Brasileira de Farmacognosia. 2013;**23**(2):239-248. DOI: 10.1590/S0102-695X2013005000017

[24] El Hadj Ali I, Guetat A, Boussaid M. A combined approach using allozymes and volatiles for the characterization of Tunisian *Thymbra capitata* (L.) Cav. (Lamiaceae). Industrial Crops and Products. 2013;**43**:477-483. DOI: 10.1016/j.indcrop.2012.07.059

[25] Saija A, Speciale A, Trombetta D, Leto C, Tuttolomondo T, La Bella S, et al. Phytochemical, ecological and antioxidant evaluation of wild Sicilian thyme: *Thymbra capitata* (L.) Cav. Chemistry and Biodiversity. 2016;**13**(12):1641-1655. DOI: 10.1002/cbdv.201600072

[26] Miguel MG, Figueiredo AC, Costa MM, Martins D, Duarte J, Barroso JG, et al. Effect of the volatile constituents isolated from *Thymus albicans*, *Th. Mastichina*, *Th. Carnosus* and *Thymbra capitata* in sunflower oil. Nahrung. 2003;**47**(6):397-402. DOI: 10.1002/food.200390089

[27] Miguel MG, Figueiredo AC, Costa MM, Martins D, Barroso JG, Pedro L. Effect of the essential volatile oils isolated from *Thymbra capitata* (L.) Cav. on olive and sunflower oils. Grasas y Aceites. 2003;**54**(3):219-225. DOI: 10.3989/gya.2003.v54.i3.234

[28] Tuttolomondo T, Dugo G, Leto C, Cicero N, Tropea A, Virga G, et al. Agronomical and chemical characterisation of *Thymbra capitata* (L.) Cav. biotypes from Sicily, Italy. Natural Product Research. 2015;**29**(14):1289-1299. DOI: 10.1080/14786419.2014.997726

[29] Miceli A, Negro C, Tommasi L. Essential oil variability in *Thymbra capitata* (L.) Cav. growing wild in southern Apulia (Italy). Biochemical Systematics and Ecology. 2006;**34**(6):528-535. DOI: 10.1016/j.bse.2005.12.010

[30] Delgado-Adámez J, Garrido M, Bote ME, Fuentes-Pérez MC, Espino J, Martín-Vertedor D. Chemical composition and bioactivity of essential oils from flower and fruit of *Thymbra capitata* and thymus species. Journal of Food Science and Technology. 2017;**54**(7):1857-1865. DOI: 10.1007/s13197-017-2617-5

[31] El Hadj Ali I, Guetat A, Boussaid M. Variation of volatiles in Tunisian populations of *Thymbra capitata* (L.) Cav. (Lamiaceae). Chemistry and Biodiversity. 2012;**9**(7):1272-1285. DOI: 10.1002/cbdv.201100344

[32] Rota MC, Herrera A, Martínez RM, Sotomayor JA, Jordán MJ. Antimicrobial activity and chemical composition of *Thymus vulgaris*, *Thymus zygis* and *Thymus hyemalis* essential oils. Food Control. 2008;**19**(7):681-687. DOI: 10.1016/j.foodcont.2007.07.007

[33] Cabo J, Crespo ME, Jimenez J, Navarro C, Risco S. Seasonal variation of essential oil yield and composition of *Thymus hyemalis*. Planta Médica. 1987;**53**(4):380-382. DOI: 10.1055/s-2006-962744

[34] Jordán MJ, Martínez RM, Cases MA, Sotomayor JA. Watering level effect on *Thymus hyemalis* Lange essential oil yield and composition. Journal of Agricultural and Food Chemistry. 2003;**51**(18):5420-5427. DOI: 10.1021/jf034335m

[35] Martínez RM, Jordán MJ, Quílez M, Sotomayor JA. Effects of edaphoclimatic conditions on *Thymus hyemalis* L. essential oil yield and composition. Journal of Essential Oil Research. 2005;**17**(6):614-618. DOI: 10.1080/10412905.2005.9699011

[36] Jordán MJ, Martínez RM, Goodner KL, Baldwin EA, Sotomayor JA. Seasonal variation of *Thymus hyemalis* Lange and Spanish *Thymus vulgaris* L. essential oils composition. The International Conference on Industrial Crops and Rural Development. 2006;**24**(3):253-263. DOI: 10.1016/j.indcrop.2006.06.011

[37] Miguel MG, Gago C, Antunes MD, Megías C, Cortés-Giraldo I, Vioque J, et al. Antioxidant and antiproliferative activities of the essential oils from *Thymbra capitata* and thymus species grown in Portugal. Evidence-based Complementary and Alternative Medicine. 2015;**2015**:1-8. DOI: 10.1155/2015/851721

[38] Aazza S, El-Guendouz S, Miguel MG, Antunes MD, Faleiro ML, Correia AI, et al. Antioxidant, anti-inflammatory and anti-hyperglycaemic activities of essential oils from *Thymbra capitata*, *Thymus albicans*, *Thymus caespititius*, *Thymus carnosus*, *Thymus lotocephalus* and *Thymus mastichina* from Portugal. Natural Product Communications. 2016;**11**(7):1029-1038

[39] Miguel MG, Antunes MD, Rohaim A, Figueiredo AF, Pedro LG, Barroso JG. Stability of fried olive and sunflower oils enriched with *Thymbra capitata* essential oil. Czech Journal of Food Sciences. 2014;**32**(1):102-108

[40] Saavedra T, Dandlen1 SA, Neves MA, Martins D, Antunes MD, Figueiredo AC, et al. Stability of olive oils during storage in the presence of *Thymbra capitata* essential oil. Stability of olive oils. Agro FOOD Industry Hi Tech. 2015;**26**(2):61-65

[41] Galego L, Almeida V, Goncalves V, Costa M, Monteiro I, Matos F, et al. Antioxidant activity of the essential

oils of *Thymbra capitata*, *Origanum vulgare*, *Thymus mastichina*, and *Calamintha baetica*. Acta Horticulturae. 2008;**765**:325-334

[42] Hortigón-Vinagre MP, Blanco J, Ruiz T, Henao F. *Thymbra capitata* essential oil prevents cell death induced by 4-hydroxy-2-nonenal in neonatal rat cardiac myocytes. Planta Medica. 2014;**80**(15):1284-1290. DOI: 10.1055/s-0034-1383051

[43] Machado DM, Alves P, Sousa C, Oliveira JM, Salgueiro L, Oliveira AP, Cerca N. Preliminary studies for the aplication of *Thymbra capitata* essential oil as potential antimicrobial agent in bacterial vaginosis. In: BioMicroWorld 2013—V International Conference on Environmental, Industrial and Applied Microbiology; 2013. pp. 502-502

[44] Machado D, Gaspar C, Palmeira-de-Oliveira A, Cavaleiro C, Salgueiro L, Martinez-de-Oliveira J, et al. *Thymbra capitata* essential oil as potential therapeutic agent against *Gardnerella vaginalis* biofilm-related infections. Future Microbiology. 2017;**12**:407-416. DOI: 10.2217/fmb-2016-0184

[45] Karampoula F, Giaouris E, Deschamps J, Doulgeraki AI, Nychas GJE, Dubois-Brissonnet F. Hydrosol of *Thymbra capitata* is a highly efficient biocide against *Salmonella enterica* Serovar *Typhimurium* biofilms. Applied and Environmental Microbiology. 2016;**82**(17):5309-5319. DOI: 10.1128/AEM.01351-16

[46] Salgueiro LR, Pinto E, Gonçalves MJ, Pina-Vaz C, Cavaleiro C, Rodrigues AG, et al. Chemical composition and antifungal activity of the essential oil of *Thymbra capitata*. Planta Medica. 2004;**70**(16):572-575. DOI: 10.1055/s-2004-827162

[47] Palmeira-de-Oliveira A, Gaspar C, Palmeira-de-Oliveira R, Silva-Dias A, Salgueiro L, Cavaleiro C, et al. The anti-candida activity of *Thymbra capitata* essential oil: Effect upon pre-formed biofilm. Journal of Ethnopharmacology. 2012;**140**(2):379-383. DOI: 10.1016/j.jep.2012.01.029

[48] Palmeira de-Oliveira A, Palmeirea de-Oliveira R, Gaspar C, Salgueiro L, Cavaleiro C, Palmeira de-Oliveira JM, et al. Association of *Thymbra capitata* essential oil and chitosan (TCCH hydrogel): A putative therapeutic tool for the treatment of vulvovaginal candidosis. Flavour and Fragrance Journal. 2013;**28**(6):354-359. DOI: 10.1002/ffj.3144

[49] Ocaña A, Reglero G. Effects of thyme extract oils (from *Thymus vulgaris*, *Thymus zygis*, and *Thymus hyemalis*) on cytokine production and gene expression of oxLDL-stimulated THP-1-macrophages. Journal of Obesity. 2012;**2012**:1-11. DOI: 10.1155/2012/104706

[50] Jennan S, Farah A, Bennani B, Fouad R, Mahjoubi F. Antibacterial and antioxidant activities of the essential oils of *Thymus hyemalis* and *Thymus bleicherianus* from Morocco. International Journal of Pharmacognosy and Phytochemistry. 2013;**28**(2):1173-1178

[51] Tepe B, Sarikurkcu C, Berk S, Alim A, Akpulat HA. Chemical composition, radical scavenging and antimicrobial activity of the essential oils of *Thymus bovei* and *Thymus hyemalis*. Records of Natural Products. 2011;**5**(3):208-220

[52] Boiraa H, Blanquer A. Environmental factors affecting chemical variability of essential oils in *Thymus piperella* L. Biochemical Systematics and Ecology. 1998;**26**(8):811-822. DOI: 10.1016/S0305-1978(98)00047-7

[53] Badi HN, Yazdani D, Ali SM, Nazari F. Effects of spacing and harvesting time on herbage yield and quality/quantity of oil in thyme,

Thymus vulgaris L. Industrial Crops and Products. 2004;**19**(3):231-236. DOI: 10.1016/j.indcrop.2003.10.005

[54] Santos FA, Rao VS. Antiinflammatory and antinociceptive effects of 1,8-cineole a terpenoid oxide present in many plant essential oils. Phytotherapy Research. 2000;**14**(4):240-244

[55] Lee BH, Annis PC, Tumaalii F, Choi WS. Fumigant toxicity of essential oils from the Myrtaceae family and 1,8-cineole against 3 major stored-grain insects. Journal of Stored Products Research. 2004;**40**(5):553-564. DOI: 10.1016/j.jspr.2003.09.001

[56] Wink M, Carey DB. Variability of quinolizidine alkaloid profiles of *Lupinus argentous* (Fabaceae) from North America. Biochemical Systematics and Ecology. 1994;**22**(7):663-669. DOI: 10.1016/0305-1978(94)90052-3

[57] Lebot V, Levesque J. Genetic control of kavalactone chemotypes in Piper methysticum cultivars. Phytochemistry. 1996;**43**(2):397-403. DOI: 10.1016/0031-9422(96)00209-9

[58] Dawidowicz AL, Olszowy M. Does antioxidant properties of the main component of essential oil reflect its antioxidant properties? The comparison of antioxidant properties of essential oils and their main components. Natural Product Research. 2014;**28**(22):1952-1963. DOI: 10.1080/14786419.2014.918121